the *Art* of
raw living
food

Also by Doreen Virtue

Books/Kits/Oracle Board

The Angel Therapy® Handbook (available October 2010)
Signs from Above (with Charles Virtue)
The Miracles of Archangel Michael
Angel Numbers 101
Solomon's Angels (a novel)
My Guardian Angel (with Amy Oscar)
Angel Blessings Candle Kit (includes booklet, CD, journal, etc.)
Thank You, Angels! (children's book with Kristina Tracy)
Healing Words from the Angels
How to Hear Your Angels
Realms of the Earth Angels
Fairies 101
Daily Guidance from Your Angels
Divine Magic
How to Give an Angel Card Reading Kit
Angels 101
Angel Guidance Board
Goddesses & Angels
Crystal Therapy (with Judith Lukomski)
Connecting with Your Angels Kit (includes booklet, CD, journal, etc.)
Angel Medicine
The Crystal Children
Archangels & Ascended Masters
Earth Angels
Messages from Your Angels
Angel Visions II
Eating in the Light (with Becky Prelitz, M.F.T., R.D.)
The Care and Feeding of Indigo Children
Healing with the Fairies
Angel Visions
Divine Prescriptions
Healing with the Angels
"I'd Change My Life If I Had More Time"
Divine Guidance
Chakra Clearing
Angel Therapy®
The Lightworker's Way
Constant Craving A–Z
Constant Craving
The Yo-Yo Diet Syndrome
Losing Your Pounds of Pain

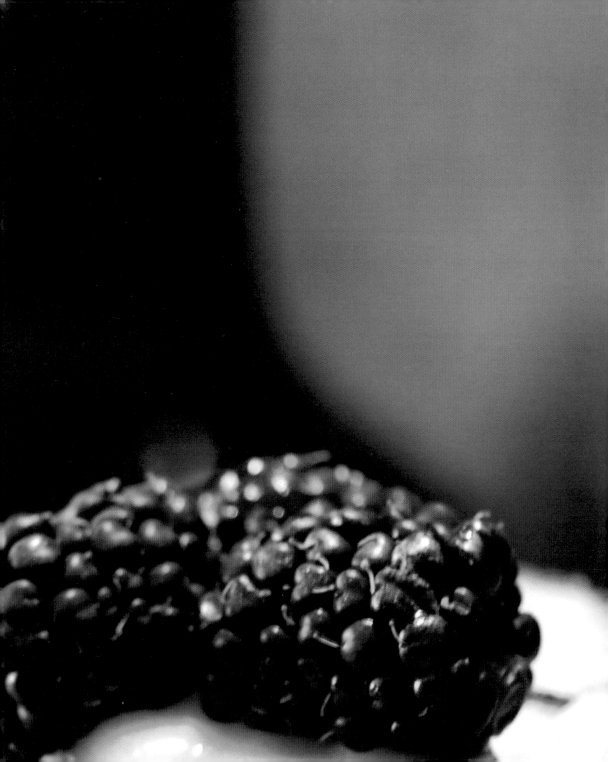

the *Art* of raw living *food*

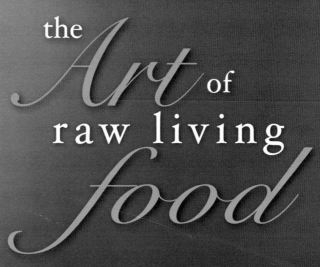

Heal Yourself and the Planet with Eco-delicious Cuisine

DOREEN VIRTUE

AND

JENNY ROSS

HAY HOUSE, INC.
Carlsbad, California • New York City
London • Sydney • Johannesburg
Vancouver • Hong Kong • New Delhi

Published and distributed in the United States by: Hay House, Inc.: www.hayhouse.com • *Published and distributed in Australia by:* Hay House Australia Pty. Ltd.: www.hayhouse.com.au • *Published and distributed in the United Kingdom by:* Hay House UK, Ltd.: www.hayhouse.co.uk • *Published and distributed in the Republic of South Africa by:* Hay House SA (Pty), Ltd.: www.hayhouse.co.za • *Distributed in Canada by:* Raincoast: www.raincoast.com • *Published in India by:* Hay House Publishers India: www.hayhouse.co.in

Editorial supervision: Jill Kramer • *Design:* Bryn Best • *All main food photography:* Kit Chan • *Thai Spring Rolls and Chocolate Ganache photos:* Ross Roca • *Additional photos:* **Dreamstime.com** • *Illustration on page viii:* Paul Kolesar (**www.paulkolesar.com**) • *Illustrations on pages 24, 42, 48, 78, 102, 132:* Lynne Taetzsch (**artbylt.com**)

Library of Congress Control Number: 2008944306

ISBN: 978-1-4019-2183-5

12 11 10 09   4 3 2 1
1st edition, September 2009

Printed in China

To my parents, Joan and Bill Hannan, who teach and exude the benefits of healthful eating. Thanks for not keeping junk food and soda in our house while I was growing up!

— Doreen

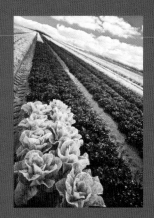

To my son, Dylan: This book and all of its contents are for you. May it help you nourish your body and soul. To my parents, Tamara and Charles Ross, who nurtured my creativity and helped me see early in my life that anything is possible. To my husband, Billy Enriquez, for his constant support from the very beginning of my journey into living foods. To Doreen for her vision, intuitive guidance, and clarity on this important work. To my business partners Kit and Shannon Chan and Mason Lazar for believing in the vision of 118 Degrees from its initial concept, and to all of the 118 team and dedicated customers who have helped make this vision a reality: we really can change the world one bite at a time!

— Jenny

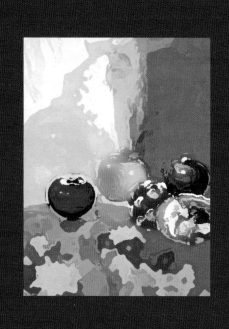

Contents

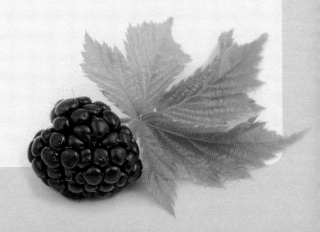

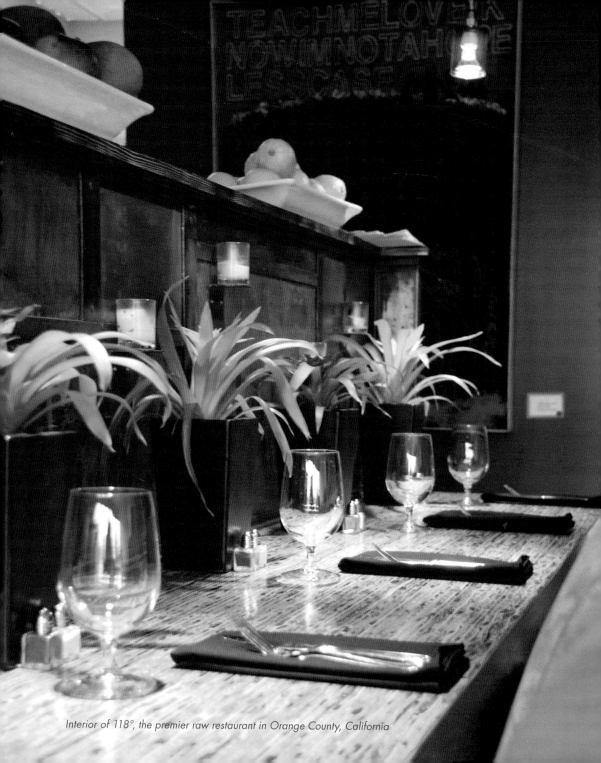

Interior of 118°, the premier raw restaurant in Orange County, California

Introduction

Around the world, a revolution is quietly occurring as people switch to "raw food" diets. *Raw food–ists*—with their youthful complexions, vibrant health, radiant skin, silky hair, and clear eyes—are inspiring others to add "living foods" into their meal plans. This new way of eating is delicious, easy, and fun . . . and it's the ultimate contribution to going green for the world's environment.

Far from just boring salads, living cuisine consists of creamy and crunchy dishes such as burritos, lasagna, pizza, sushi, and apple pie—all cleverly created from fruits, vegetables, nuts, seeds, and sprouted grains. Restaurants devoted to raw food are popping up internationally, and celebrities are touting its fountain-of-youth benefits.

The philosophy behind raw food is both nutritional and spiritual. Fresh produce contains living and healthful enzymes, which are killed when it's cooked above 118 degrees Fahrenheit. By profession, I (Jenny) am the owner and executive chef of a living-foods restaurant called 118 Degrees in Costa Mesa, California. I know that the enzymes, vitamins, minerals, fiber, and pure energy within raw food can heal and detoxify the body. Many formerly ill people credit their raw diets with saving their lives.

The highly processed, cooked foods of the Standard American Diet (SAD) contribute to lethargy, obesity, and disease. Just by adding a small percentage of raw food to the SAD, people lose weight and feel better.

Raw food also answers the call to "go green," since it supports sustainable organic farming; and as a vegetarian diet, it's a cruelty-free lifestyle.

Those who "go raw" find that their intuitive and psychic abilities immediately increase because the life-force spirit of food supports the soul's natural gifts. In fact, I (Doreen) have been a vegan since 1996, consuming 80 to 90 percent raw food (I even went 100 percent raw for one year!); and when I first adopted this diet, I noticed a huge increase in my energy and psychic abilities. As a former psychotherapist, I'm also aware of the importance of a healthful diet in maintaining mental and physical well-being.

In 2004, *Medical News Today* reported raw food as one of the seven most popular diets in the world. **Google.com** has 1.7 million sites devoted to this style of eating. Although there are at least 100 raw-food restaurants in the world, most people prepare their own dishes from recipes such as those within this book.

Raw Living Foods

We're often asked to define *raw foods* by people who wonder if we're talking about uncooked meat or fish, as in sushi. By "raw living foods," we mean vegetarian meals that mimic traditional Italian, Mexican, Asian, and other cultures' dishes . . . all composed of cleverly formed uncooked vegetables, fruits, nuts, nut milks, sprouted grains, and herbs.

Raw living food goes beyond salads to bring you interesting variations on ways to enjoy your vegetables. To maintain ingredients' optimal nutrients—such as vitamins, minerals, and enzymes (which cooking destroys)—they are never heated above 118 degrees.

This type of food promotes health and life. As creatures composed of more than 60 percent water, we require living nutrition to maintain vitality and health. So, raw living food has been known to:

- Increase stamina
- Improve mental focus and clarity
- Lower cholesterol
- Reverse "life-threatening" diseases and conditions
- Promote healthy skin and hair growth
- Improve vision

- Create a youthful, glowing complexion
- Revitalize overworked organs
- Prevent osteoporosis
- Maintain longevity
- Uplift and stabilize moods and emotions
- Increase spiritual awareness and gifts

The more fresh, living foods we consume daily, the healthier our minds and bodies will be. This is something that science has known for decades. In 1930, Swiss scientists discovered that immediately after we consume cooked foods, our bodies increase the number of white blood cells in the bloodstream. This process doesn't occur after eating raw food—it only comes in response to the unhealthful properties in the cooked variety. The number of white blood cells increased significantly especially in response to processed cooked food, such as white flour or white rice.

In addition, cookware itself presents health dangers. Nonstick coating gives off toxic fumes, aluminum leaches into food, and plastic (as in spatulas) that's microwaved or heated unleashes harmful chemicals. If you must cook, always use stainless-steel, glass, or wooden cookware.

The Healthful Truth about Raw Living Foods

Our bodies need vitamins and minerals for basic and optimal health, and the best source for these nutrients is fresh fruits and vegetables. Here are some of the beneficial properties and contents of raw food:

— **Enzymes.** Uncooked foods contain *enzymes*, which are proteins that are catalysts for digestion, immune-system functioning, energy production, and brain activity. Since heat destroys one of the most vital types and changes all enzymes' structure, cooking diminishes the vital nutrients in your meals! Cooked food is therefore difficult to digest, puts undue stress on your pancreas, and sits in your body longer. Raw food digests in one-half to one-third the time of its cooked counterpart.

— **Protein.** Cooking destroys at least one-half of food's available protein—the building block of muscular growth and regeneration! Vegetables, fruits, nuts, and legumes contain more than sufficient protein to fuel healthy bodies. In addition, since raw living food is vegan, you avoid animal-based proteins, which studies have linked to cancer, osteoporosis, and other health concerns.

— **pH balance.** Raw living foods also help you maintain a homeostatic balance of alkaline and acid, which increasing numbers of studies link to health, youthfulness, and longevity. The Standard American Diet creates an extremely acidic environment for the body, making it more susceptible to disease and degeneration. In contrast, most raw and unprocessed fruits and vegetables have a healthful alkaline effect on the body.

— **Vitamins and minerals.** Cooking destroys 50 to 80 percent of vitamins and minerals in foods and half of the antioxidants and carotenoids, thereby reducing the nutritional value of your meals. For example, it destroys 50 to 96 percent of B vitamins—including 97 percent of folic acid and 72 percent of biotin—and up to 80 percent of vitamin C.

A 2006 Louisiana State University study examined the diets of more than 10,000 men and women. Researchers found that those who consumed the most raw vegetables and salads had significantly higher blood-serum levels of vitamins C and E, folic acid, and carotenoids. The study concluded that these nutrients were well absorbed from a diet of salad and raw vegetables.

Another study conducted in Finland in 1995 found that raw living food–ists had significantly higher blood levels of vitamins C and E and beta-carotene, even when they weren't consuming nutritional supplements.

— **Water.** Since our bodies are 60 to 70 percent water, we need to hydrate throughout the day. Cooking effectively *dehydrates* food.

— **Oils.** The natural oils in food are denatured through the cooking process, rendering it more difficult to digest and utilize. This happens as the molecular structure of the oil is changed during exposure to high heat, making it literally a poison in the body.

The Physical, Mental, and Spiritual Benefits of Raw Living Foods

As you incorporate more raw living foods into your daily diet, you'll soon discover that it's a lifestyle and not just an eating plan. That's why some raw food–ists become a little fanatical—they're models for the many emotional and spiritual benefits of eating uncooked foods. These benefits include the following:

— **Optimal daily health.** A feeling of peace, tranquility, and harmony accompanies our bodies when they're in a balanced state of optimal nutrition. It's easier to get going in the morning, with more energy throughout the day and mental clarity for better performance at home and at work.

A 1985 study reported in *Southern Medical Journal* found that a raw-food diet significantly reduced blood pressure, resulted in weight loss, and led 80 percent of participants to abstain from alcohol and cigarette consumption.

Other studies show beneficial health effects for those who have rheumatoid arthritis and fibromyalgia. And because raw vegan food is completely cholesterol free, it's a heart-healthy diet.

Raw-food eating brings benefits rapidly as well! A 1992 Finish study discovered statistically significant health improvement among chronically ill people when they switched to an all-raw-vegetable diet *for just one week!* An infamous experiment called the China Study found that tumors grew in rats fed a high-animal-fat diet, yet researchers discovered that the tumors reversed when the animal fat was removed or replaced with plant fats (such as vegetable oils, avocados, or nuts). They also linked breast cancer and diabetes to the consumption of animal-based protein. In addition, a 1990 German study found that a raw vegan diet significantly boosted the immune system.

— **Ecological friendliness and freedom from cruelty.** Any form of vegetarianism reduces the pollution and cruelty connected to animals raised for meat, fur, or leather. Compared to meat, dairy, eggs, and other animal products, a diet of vegetables and fruit (especially organic and locally grown varieties) means less water consumption, carbon footprints, air pollution, and toxic chemical runoff into waterways.

— **Weight loss.** When you stop eating high-fat animal products, you automatically lose weight. A 1999 German study found that women shed an average of 26 pounds and men an average of 22 pounds after going on a raw-food diet. A similar study conducted in Finland in 1993 found that raw-food participants lost an average of 9 percent of their body weight.

— **Long-term health.** Eating a raw-living-food diet is preventive medicine at its best. A healthy, balanced living-foods diet can stave off disease in the body, ultimately reducing risks of cancer, heart disease, diabetes, poor vision, and arthritis.

— **Beauty.** Healthy hair, skin, and fingernails; optimal weight management; and sound immune function lead to all aspects of beauty, inside and out. The density of vitamins and nutrients available in raw fruits and vegetables supports a beautiful body and mind.

But What about Protein?

Some people worry that a raw vegan diet won't provide sufficient protein for their bodies' needs. Even if you're not worried, your family and friends may express this concern after you adopt a living-foods lifestyle.

The American Dietetic Association in a 2003 position statement said that "appropriately planned vegetarian diets are healthful [and] nutritionally adequate." This means that you'll still need to be cognizant of eating enough plant-based protein for your body's individual needs.

According to Gabriel Cousens, M.D., an author of books about raw living foods, certain people do need a higher percentage of protein (up to 50 percent) in their diets. He calls such individuals "fast oxidizers" and "parasympathetics"; and recommends that they supplement their raw vegan diets with high-protein sea vegetables such as blue-green algae, spirulina, and chlorella (which contain up to 70 percent protein), as well as leafy vegetables like kale.

If you look at our primate cousins, you'll see that many have very adequate and healthful diets that are completely vegetarian. Gorillas eat 95 percent green vegetation and 5 percent fruit . . . and they have no problem being big and strong!

A comparison of the amino-acid content of lamb meat and kale shows that the hearty cabbage actually yields higher percentages of this protein component. In addition, most raw food–ists supplement their diets daily with high-protein nuts and seeds.

As we mentioned, the famous China Study discovered that animal protein was the key trigger mechanism in the growth of tumors within laboratory rats. The lead scientist wrote that animal protein in the diet "proved to be so powerful in its effect that we could turn on and turn off cancer growth simply by changing the level [of animal protein] consumed."

A (Very) Few Drawbacks to a Raw Diet

With all of these benefits, you may wonder if there are any *negative* effects of eating a raw living diet. To keep this book objective and truthful, here are some downsides that are possible but not probable:

— **Dental issues.** If you're eating a lot of fruit, it's important to brush your teeth frequently. Tooth decay is one possible outcome of consuming too much fruit without any additionally balancing plant-based fats.

— **Sensitive emotions and relationship changes.** A raw diet cleanses your system of any toxic chemicals that formerly played a part in controlling and dulling your emotions. Many people report that eating a diet that's free of toxins makes them hypersensitive to the emotions and personalities of those around them. The reality is that since your body no longer has to remove food toxins, you're more open to experiencing other parts of life. For some, this can open the door to in-depth emotional healing.

You may also find that people you formerly enjoyed are now difficult for you to be with. On the other hand, you'll very likely attract healthy new friends and enjoy an increase in accurate intuition. You'll also experience more of the true essence of who you are. Once your cells are functioning optimally, a whole new world of love and light is available to you.

— **Weight gain or loss.** If you eat too many fats from nuts, nut butters, avocados, and olives, you're likely to gain weight on a raw-food diet. Conversely, some people lose too much weight, and studies have found that women skip menstrual periods on low-calorie raw-food diets. So do pay attention to your fat and caloric consumption, as well as your weight, menstrual cycles (if you're a woman), and general vitality level. Balance is a key component of success when making any dietary change.

— **Detoxification effects.** The purifying process of a raw-food diet can trigger a detoxification of all the fried food, sugar, white flour, and preservatives of your former diet. Normal detoxification effects include nausea, skin issues, and bowel changes. Fortunately, these are temporary and last only until your body becomes accustomed to the higher-quality raw-food diet.

— **Vitamin B_{12} deficiencies.** All vegans are prone to this deficiency, which is easily overcome by taking B_{12} sublingual supplements. One study also found that vegans who eat seaweed and sea vegetables have sufficient B_{12} levels.

— **Pesticides.** Unless you're eating organic vegetables and fruits, there are pesticide residues on the produce in a raw-food diet. (However, medical doctor, author, and raw-food proponent Gabriel Cousens points out that "normal" foods contain many more pathogenic microorganisms such as fungi and mycotoxins than the average vegan meal. For example, the average meat eater consumes 750 million to 1 billion pathogenic microorganisms per meal, compared to 500 for vegans.)

Detoxification with Raw Living Foods

Our bodies absorb many toxins from the environment. The average American comes into contact with 133 toxins daily through pollution, food, manufactured cleansers, and synthetic products. The body is powerful and can completely regenerate if nourished correctly.

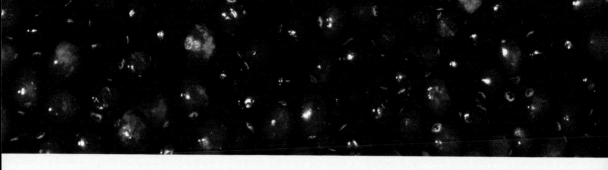

Living foods are naturally detoxifying, and therefore your body can effectively isolate toxins within itself and properly eliminate them, leading to greater health, clarity, and longevity. When you begin eating a predominantly raw diet, you may experience detoxification effects.

Here are some raw foods that have powerful detoxifying properties:

Fruits for Detoxification

- **Lemon, lime, pineapple, and grapefruit:** Act as solvents, which are good for cleaning the liver and gallbladder. Pineapple contains the enzyme bromelain, which helps in healing and digesting protein.

- **Apple:** A powerful digestive cleanser.

- **Cranberry:** A diuretic and kidney cleanser that detoxes the urinary tract, and also draws out chemicals and toxins.

- **Watermelon:** A diuretic to flush out any water-based toxins or eliminate fluid retention from a high-sodium diet.

Vegetables for Detoxification

- **Greens**—such as kale, spinach, and parsley—are healing, cleansing, calming, and centering.

- **Sea vegetables** are high in B vitamins.

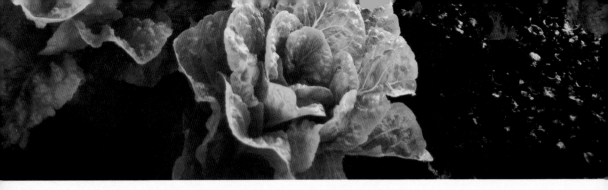

Vegetable- and Fruit-Juice Home Remedies

Here are delicious raw living juice recommendations to support your health:

- **Cold fighters:** carrot, lemon, radish, ginger, garlic
- **Immune boosters:** carrot, celery, parsley, garlic
- **Stress relievers:** carrot, celery, kale, parsley, broccoli, tomato
- **Detoxifiers:** apple, beet, cucumber, ginger
- **Antioxidant boosts:** carrot, orange, green pepper, ginger
- **Liver cleaner:** wheatgrass
- **Digestive aids:** pineapple, papaya

Raw-Living-Food Kitchen Necessities

Before we begin with the recipes, let's look at the basics you'll want to keep in your kitchen to make your food preparation painless and enjoyable. This is a guide meant to help direct you to the finest ingredients to share with your family and friends.

— **Apple-cider vinegar:** Cider vinegar has amazing healing properties and can be used to create a variety of dressings and sauces for your raw dishes. Spectrum and Bragg make beautiful cider vinegars that stay high quality in the refrigerator indefinitely.

— **Buckwheat groats:** High in protein and a handy ingredient for dehydrated or fresh recipes, these hulled grains are easy to sprout and are found in the bulk section of most natural-products retailers.

— **Celtic sea salt:** Sea salt in moderation is great as a ga
enhancer. It's important that it be used instead of table salt to avoi
and processing in the latter. Celtic sea salt is sun dried and can be
health-food stores. Gold Mine and Herbamare (which contains dried ve
seasoning) are excellent brands.

— **Cinnamon:** This universal spice is one we use in many dishes. Fresh sticks or organic powdered cinnamon is the best choice.

— **Dried herb-blend seasoning:** Italian, Mediterranean, and Spanish are nice herb blends to make a quick dish more flavorful in seconds. At your local health-food store, look for organic blends with nothing added.

— **Gourmet oils:** Avocado, sesame, hazelnut, macadamia, and truffle oils are some of our favorites. Gourmet oils greatly enhance the flavor in many dressings and sauces and are great poured over salad and pasta alone. Choose raw or cold-pressed (extra-virgin) varieties.

— **Himalayan salt:** This pink salt from the Himalayan mountains tastes incredible and can be used on its own as a supplement or added to dishes for superior flavor and optimal nutrition. Many health-food and online stores sell this item.

— **Miso:** Miso paste enhances flavor and creates a salty taste for those with sodium sensitivities. Always look for aged miso, and the brown-rice type is preferable. This product is fermented and can be found at most health-food stores. Once opened, it lasts several days refrigerated.

— **Nuts and seeds:** It's always good to keep raw nuts—such as almonds (helps keep alkalinity in the body), Brazil nuts (high in selenium), pine nuts, and macadamia nuts—and seeds in the kitchen to create with on a whim. These are easy for the body to digest and can be used alone or in combination to create amazing dishes. Pumpkin seeds can be readily sprouted and make a great seed cheese. Flaxseed is also essential and comes in a golden or dark brown color.

— **Olive oil:** Use an organic first- or cold-pressed extra-virgin (or "raw") olive oil in your recipes. Premium varieties create an amazing flavor in dressings, sauces, and spreads. Olive oil should be kept in a dark glass bottle to block the light and prevent the contents from becoming rancid. Store it in a dark, cool place. Bariani and Oliflix are excellent brands to use in meal preparation. Bariani is stone-ground to guarantee no heat during the pressing process.

— **Psyllium husk:** This is a great thickening agent in a raw kitchen, with a variety of uses in wraps, pies, and puddings. It's often found in the supplement section at your local health-food store, and keeps indefinitely in an airtight container.

— **Raw agave nectar:** This is one of the best sweeteners for raw-foods preparation because it's low on the glycemic index and safe for diabetics and those with sugar sensitivities. Agave comes from a cactus flower and is extracted at low temperatures. It's readily available in health-food and online stores.

— **Raw cacao beans:** Raw chocolate is great in desserts and other savory dishes, or when used as a garnish.

— **Raw carob powder:** Derived from the carob pod, this is a nice alternative to chocolate and is rich in protein. This powder can be found in raw form at most health-food stores and can be stored in an airtight container indefinitely.

— **Vanilla bean:** Vanilla adds a nice soothing, mellow flavor to desserts and some entrée dishes.

— **Young Thai coconuts:** "Nature's water"! The liquid from a young Thai coconut is the purest on the planet and full of electrolytes to hydrate the body. We use the flesh of this fruit in many desserts and wraps as well as breakfast items. It's found at Asian markets and health-food stores.

Tools for Raw-Food Preparation

— **High-powered blender:** A Vita-Mix blender is our recommendation here. It has a strong motor, and the design of the container allows you to use a plunger for the harder-to-blend nut and seed cheeses. In some recipes in this book, you'll specifically read "high-powered blender" in the directions. Others not requiring the extra speed or power of a Vita-Mix simply call for a "blender," which means the ordinary kitchen appliance.

— **Cutting board:** A quality wood cutting board is preferable. Bamboo is quite nice.

— **Dehydrator:** Essential for preparing crunchy and crispy crackers and dried fruits, as well as marinating vegetables and creating wraps of all sorts.

— **Food processor:** Important for making cookies, crusts, pâtés, and salsas.

— **Garnishing machines:** Great to add texture, presentation, and excitement to even the simplest salads. Machines include the spiral vegetable slicer, the mandoline, and the Saladacco.

— **Knives:** You'll need sharp knives with good edges that are designed for fruits and vegetables.

— **Mixing bowls:** Glass or stainless steel is preferable. Avoid aluminum, which leaches into food.

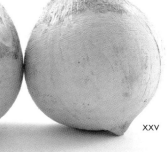

A Five-Day Sample Meal Plan

When you're embarking on any new eating pattern, it's important to remember that old habits and emotions may have a tendency to knock you off course. Please be gentle with yourself as you take this journey.

After just five short days of a living-foods diet, you should experience increased energy and enjoy greater mental clarity, your skin could begin to develop a healthful glow, and you may feel elated and more relaxed. These and many other benefits are available to you every day as you move toward greater freedom with your food choices and begin to discover all that nature has intended for your health and wellness.

We recommend that as you enjoy this five-day meal plan, you take some time to reflect, journal, and stretch to enhance the healing benefits of your raw-living-foods lifestyle. All of the suggested meals incorporate recipes from this book (the names of which are capitalized).

During every day's meals, you'll find a healthful amount of protein, fresh vegetables, vitamins, minerals, and other nutrients. Be sure to drink at least eight glasses of water throughout the day. In the morning and evening, it may be helpful to do some affirmations about your food, such as: "I enjoy vibrant health as a result of my exceptional food choices."

Day 1

Breakfast: Merry Monkey Smoothie

Early lunch: Taco Salad

Lunch: Yogi Juice;
1 handful soaked almonds
or Sicilian Flax Crackers with fresh
vegetables (try sliced tomato, fresh basil,
and chopped spinach)

Dinner: Topaz Pizza

Day 2

Breakfast: Supergreen Smoothie

Early lunch: Shiitake Salad

Lunch: Apple-Lemon-Ginger Juice;
almond butter on fresh apple
or sprouted-grain bread

Dinner: Asian Infusion

Day 3

Breakfast: Peaches-and-Cream Smoothie

Early lunch: Curry Cones

Lunch: Green Juice;
small green salad
with Miso Dressing or
Sicilian Flax Crackers
with Green Guacamole

Dinner: Heirloom-Squash Samosa

Day 4

Breakfast: Chocolate Supreme Smoothie

Early lunch: Deviled Tomatoes; Caesar Salad

Lunch: Pineapple Power Juice;
fresh vegetables with
Almond Cheese, or
fresh fruit with Vanilla Sauce

Dinner: Living Lasagna

Day 5

Breakfast: Avocado Whip Smoothie

Early lunch: Shiitake Sushi Rolls

Lunch: Beet Magic Juice;
Raw Ramen Bowl

Dinner: Clayudas

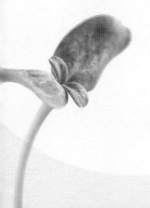

Each day you're consuming a rainbow of fruits and vegetables, nuts and seeds, and in some cases, sprouted grains.

It's important to balance a raw diet by alternating your foods and enjoying at least 50 to 70 percent fresh fruits and vegetables (not dehydrated) to hydrate your body. A common pitfall in the beginning of a living-foods diet is consuming too many unsprouted nuts and seeds and dehydrated foods without getting enough fresh, living cuisine. This is why we suggest at least one salad, juice, or smoothie in your daily diet.

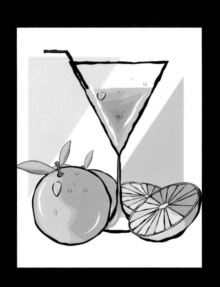

Chapter One

Drinks and Smoothies

Smoothies, juices, nut milks, elixirs, and tonics are part of the living-foods juice bar that is eternally flowing with fresh ideas for optimal nutrition, energy, and vibrant life. At the 118 Degrees restaurant, we incorporate several superfoods into our juice and smoothie mixtures.

Feel free to experiment with these recipes, adding different superfoods and fruits based on what is in your cabinet, how your body is feeling, and any special needs you may have. Smoothies and juices are a great way to put a lot of dense nutrient value into your daily diet. During the period of transition to a living-foods diet, many people do very well by having a superfood smoothie for breakfast.

Ensuring that your body receives nutrients in the morning activates your brain, lymphatic systems, and vital organs. This detoxifies your bloodstream and compels you to make better food choices throughout the whole day. Try it for yourself and see!

Superfood Guide

These supplements boost the nutritional value of your smoothies and also add delicious flavor. Here is a list of the vitamins and minerals they contain, among other properties:

- **Spirulina:** Contains 60 percent protein, as well as phytonutrients such as beta-carotene, chlorophyll, GLA essential fatty acid, vitamin B_{12} and B complex, and iron.

- **E$_3$Live:** Contains three to five times more chlorophyll than wheatgrass—plus vitamin B_{12}; essential fatty acids, including omega-3s; and 22 amino acids.

- **Maca root:** Contains more than 55 phytochemicals known to elevate mood, improve endurance, and enhance blood circulation; also high in amino acids and B vitamins, including B_{12}.

- **Hemp protein:** Rich in omega-3, omega-6, and omega-9—essential amino acids known for muscle-building ability—and high in antioxidants.

- **Bee pollen, propolis, or royal jelly:** Gets high antioxidant score; is energy enhancing; and contains dense nutrients, including omega-3s and B-complex vitamins. Some vegans don't use substances from bees because they're technically an animal by-product, so this is an optional ingredient depending upon your beliefs.

- **Chia seeds:** Contain calcium, slow down the conversion of carbohydrates into sugar, and prolong hydration. High-energy and endurance food.

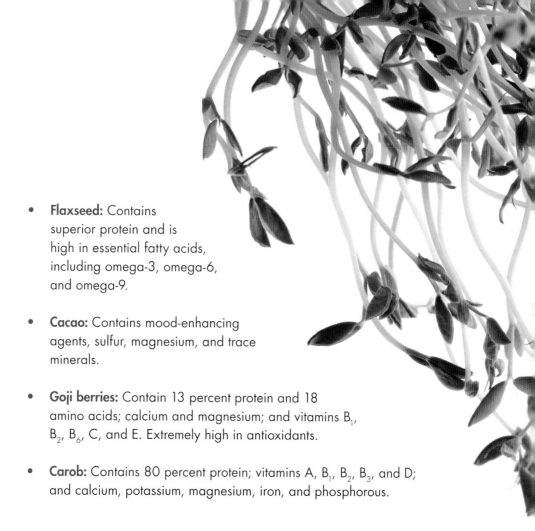

- **Flaxseed:** Contains superior protein and is high in essential fatty acids, including omega-3, omega-6, and omega-9.

- **Cacao:** Contains mood-enhancing agents, sulfur, magnesium, and trace minerals.

- **Goji berries:** Contain 13 percent protein and 18 amino acids; calcium and magnesium; and vitamins B_1, B_2, B_6, C, and E. Extremely high in antioxidants.

- **Carob:** Contains 80 percent protein; vitamins A, B_1, B_2, B_3, and D; and calcium, potassium, magnesium, iron, and phosphorous.

Juices

— STRAWBERRY-KIWI JUICE —

This juice is packed with vitamin C and is great for kids. A glass of it is better than most vitamin-supplement counterparts and can be easily absorbed in the digestive system. Kiwis by weight have 500 times more vitamin C than oranges!

4 kiwis
8 freshly picked strawberries
1 apple

Prepare kiwis for juicing by cutting off fuzzy skin and discarding it. Rinse the strawberries and remove the stems. Prepare the apple by cutting into 4 even pieces and discarding the core. Juice all ingredients. For a fun presentation, put in a shaker and add 2 pieces of ice. Shake well and pour into martini glass.

— CLEANSING COCKTAIL—

Fruit and vegetable juices are powerfully cleansing for the body. Juice fasts are great ways to give your body a break during the year and allow natural detoxification to occur. You can enjoy a cleansing cocktail every day to start it off right and push toxins out of the body.

2 apples
1 lemon
½ inch ginger root

2 stalks celery
2 cups spinach
2 oz. wheatgrass or E_3Live

Prepare apples by rinsing well and cutting them off the core into 4 pieces each. Peel lemon and discard skin. Peel ginger using vegetable peeler. Rinse celery and spinach well. Juice the apples, lemon, ginger, celery, and spinach by alternating each ingredient. Add in wheatgrass or E_3Live, and stir well.

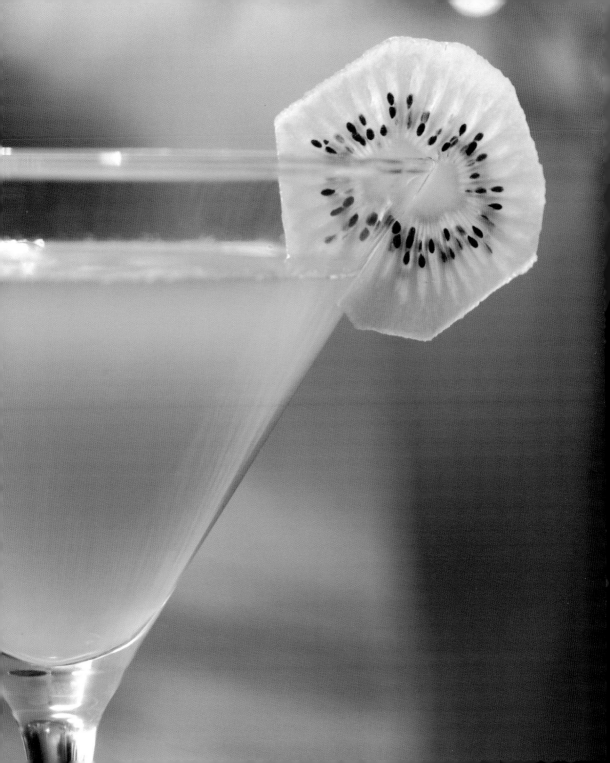

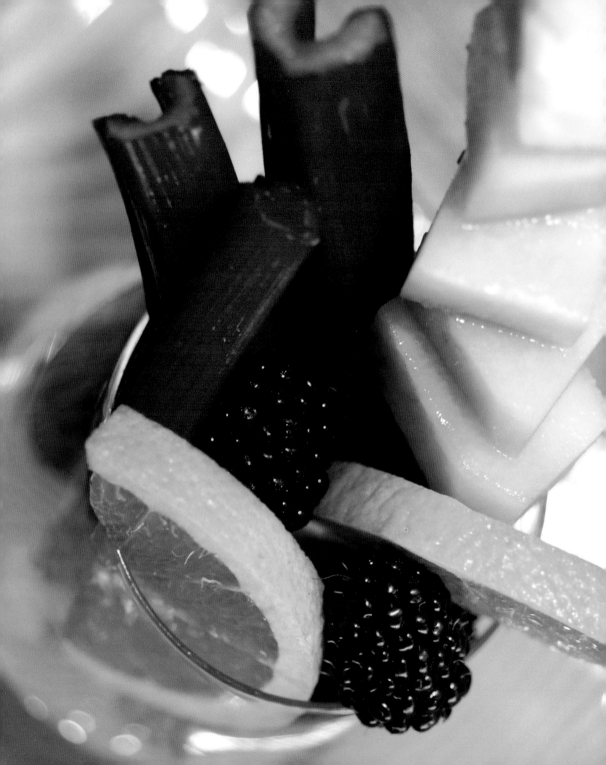

— RAINBOW-LIGHT JUICE —

Just as rainbows are created from a broad spectrum of light, this juice is a beautiful combination of energy from organic fruits and vegetables, designed to feed the body more than 133 trace minerals, nutrients, and vitamins.

2 oranges
6 blueberries
½ honeydew melon

3 leaves red chard
2 tsp. bee pollen (optional)
2 tsp. agave nectar (optional)

Prepare berries and chard by rinsing well, and set aside. Peel orange, and cut rind from honeydew melon and discard. Juice oranges, berries, chard, and melon; then pour juice into blender. Blend in bee pollen (optional, or substitute with maca-root or mesquite powder) and agave as desired. Enjoy this drink any time of the day for a quick pick-me-up!

— YOGI JUICE —

Yoga is an excellent way to open the pathways of the body and realign mind, body, and spirit. This high-energy, high-vibration drink is a favorite of our yoga students at 118 and is universally enjoyed as a refreshing juice with minerals and protein.

2 oranges
6 freshly picked strawberries
1 tsp. maca-root powder
1 lemon

2 tsp. bee pollen (optional)
1 tsp. agave nectar (optional)

Prepare citrus by rinsing and peeling. Prepare berries for juicing by cutting off stems. Juice orange, strawberries, and lemon; then place mixture in blender. Blend well with maca root, bee pollen (optional, or substitute mesquite powder or additional maca root), and agave if desired. Serve in a tall glass with berry-puree topping!

— BEET MAGIC JUICE —

Beets are great for lowering cholesterol, working directly on the heart and other circulatory systems of the body. This drink is affectionately known as "Doug's Drink" at the 118 restaurant. Doug is a regular customer of ours who has been "juicing" with great results for more than 30 years. He swears by beets and their magical powers to heal the body. Enjoy!

2 beets
2 apples
1 carrot

Prepare all ingredients for juicing by rinsing well. Cut apples off the core into 4 pieces each. Cut the top off carrot, and peel beets. Juice all ingredients by alternating pieces of carrot, apple, and beet for a more enjoyable juicing experience.

— PINEAPPLE POWER JUICE —

Pineapple contains the powerful enzyme bromelain, which is especially good for the entire digestive tract. This is a great juice for intestinal cleansing and is a perfect cooldown on a warm summer day. It can also be blended with ice to make a virgin cocktail for any special occasion!

½ medium pineapple
1 mango
1 orange

½ cup young Thai coconut water
2 tsp. agave nectar (optional)

Prepare all ingredients (except coconut) for juicing by cutting off and discarding skins. Juice, and add young Thai coconut water to the mixture. Pour liquid into shaker with a cube of ice and agave, and shake well to serve.

Slushy-style: Blend ½ cup ice and juice mixture, and pour into tumblers. Garnish with orange zest or pineapple spear.

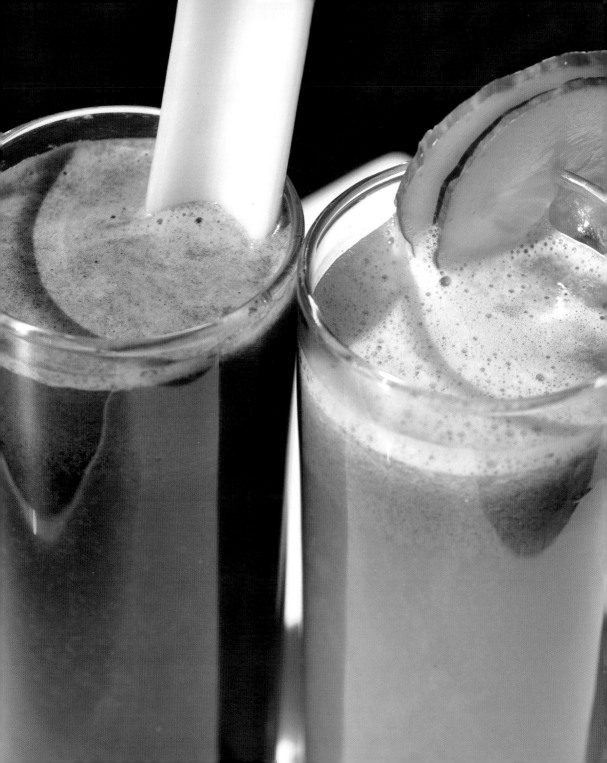

— APPLE-TWIST JUICE —

Apples have unique enzymes in their juice that work quite effectively on gallstones and liver blockages and are widely recommended during cleansing detoxes. On a daily basis, apples provide a great source of vitamins and nutrients. (When juicing them, always leave the skins on, as they contain vital nutrients.) Try the cider variation of this recipe for a great holiday treat!

    2 apples
    ¼ orange
    2 pears

Prepare all ingredients for juicing by rinsing well. Cut apples and pears off the core into 4 pieces each. Peel orange and discard skin. Juice all ingredients and enjoy!

Cider-style: During holiday season, add 1 tsp. agave nectar, 1 tsp. cinnamon, and a dash of nutmeg for a great apple cider. Gently warm on the stove using a thermometer or in the dehydrator at 110° for 2 hours.

— SPICY TOMATO JUICE —

Vegetable juice acts as a building block in the body and is good for muscles, connective fibers, and tissues. Spicy tomato juice is especially beneficial for the kidneys and for liver function. This powerful drink is high in minerals and hydrating for the body . . . great before or after a workout!

    2 tomatoes   1 carrot
    3 stalks celery   ⅛ cup cilantro or parsley
    ½ beet   1 tsp. cayenne pepper

Prepare all ingredients for juicing by washing well to remove any dirt. Cut tomatoes into quarters, and peel skin from beet. Chop the top off carrot. Juice all ingredients (except cayenne). Stir in cayenne, and garnish juice with celery or an apple round.

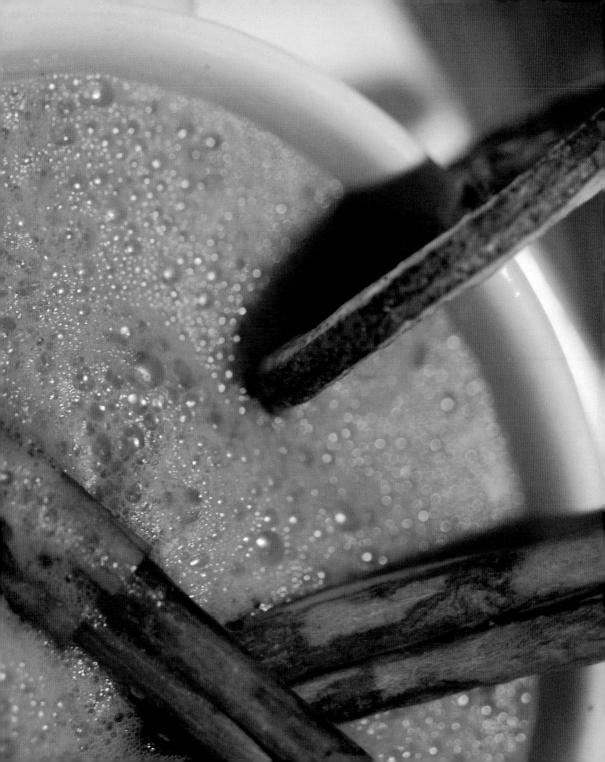

— TROPICAL-TWIST JUICE —

The tropics are known for clear water, warm breezes, and an overall feeling of blissful sweetness. Try this juice anytime you have a hunger for total relaxation.

¼ medium pineapple
1 kaffir lime
1 kiwi

1 mango
½ cup young Thai coconut water
2 tsp. agave nectar (optional)

Prepare all ingredients (except coconut) for juicing by cutting off and discarding skins. Juice all ingredients, and place in blender. Add coconut water and agave. Blend well until froth appears. Pour into glass, and garnish with an umbrella or zest from kaffir lime.

— GREEN JUICE —

Why "green"? The unique combination of chlorophyll and protein derived from the greens in this drink is the quickest way for the body to absorb these vital nutrients. This vegetable juice is also low in sugar and high in electrolytes, aiding the muscles and joints in recovery.

4 leaves kale
3 stalks celery
½ hothouse cucumber
2 cups spinach
1 apple

Prepare greens for juicing by washing well. Cut apple off the core into 4 pieces. Juice ingredients in an alternating pattern—leafy greens, cucumber, leafy greens, celery, and so on—until all are thoroughly juiced. Enjoy this elixir after yoga or any other activity for a burst of revitalizing energy.

— KALE CRAZY JUICE —

Vitamin packed and full of protein, this spicy green juice will make you feel like you can fly! Kale is especially high in iron and protein and is good for building muscles. This drink is a favorite of athletes and scholars alike, as it wakes up the mind and provides an ability to concentrate intensely.

6 leaves kale	2 oz. E_3Live BrainON
3 stalks celery	1 pear

Prepare all ingredients for juicing by rinsing well (except E_3Live). Cut pear into 4 pieces and discard core. Juice kale, celery, and pear; then pour liquid into shaker and add E_3Live and 2 cubes of ice. Shake well. Pour mixture into a highball glass and enjoy through a twisty straw if you like!

— APPLE-LEMON-GINGER JUICE —

This is a powerfully detoxifying drink! Apple-Lemon-Ginger also delivers a potent energetic jump start to any day and can be enhanced by adding cayenne pepper to further open up the lymphatic system.

2 apples (Fuji and Braeburn are our favorites!)	½ inch ginger root
2 lemons	2 tsp. cayenne pepper (optional)

Prepare ginger root for juicing by peeling the outside skin with a vegetable peeler. Prepare apples by slicing into 4 equal parts around the core. Cut or peel the skins from the lemons and discard. Begin by juicing lemons and the slices from one of the apples; and then add the ginger, then the rest of apple, until all ingredients are well juiced.

When juice-fasting, this drink is a great way to open up the chest and the vital organs of this area and promote blood circulation throughout the body. We recommend that you double this recipe during all-liquid diets and enjoy first thing in the morning.

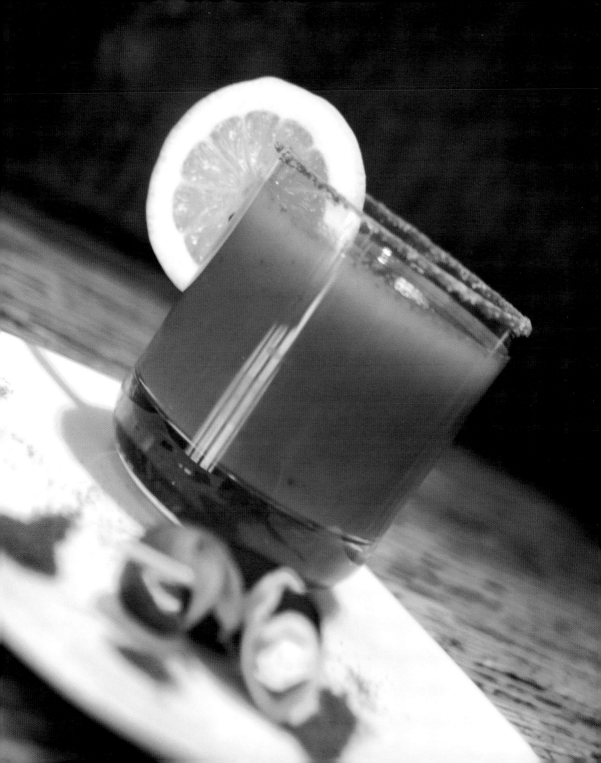

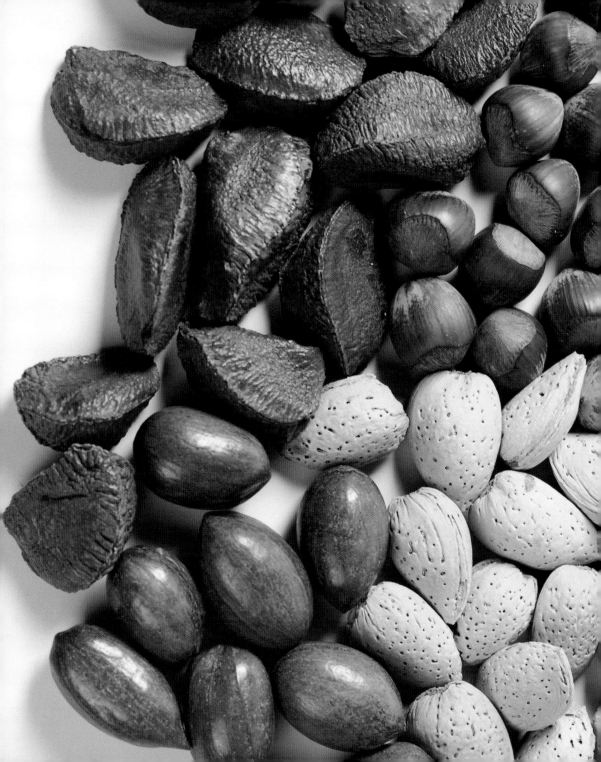

Nut Milks

When it comes to nut milk, the sky's the limit—almonds, Brazil nuts, coconuts, macadamias, hemp seeds, sesame seeds . . . and more! Here are a couple of our favorites and a basic technique for making your own.

— ALMOND MILK —

This is a rich and flavorful drink enjoyed by those who love a glass of cold milk by itself! Almonds are also naturally alkalizing, and this milk can help clear up an acid stomach.

4 cups almonds (soaked 8 hours) 1 pinch sea salt 1 Tbsp. mesquite powder
4 cups mineralized water 1 Tbsp. raw honey
1 Tbsp. vanilla 1 pinch cinnamon

Rinse almonds well and drain. Blend 2 cups soaked almonds with 2 cups water. Strain mixture through your choice of nut-milk bag or cheesecloth. Repeat. Save nut meat for other recipes, stored in refrigerated airtight container. (Use within 24 hours.) Combine freshly squeezed nut milk, vanilla, sea salt, honey, cinnamon, and mesquite in blender and lightly blend. Chill and enjoy!

—BRAZIL-NUT MILK —

Brazil nuts are high in selenium, a mineral compound that can be difficult to find in food but is essential for our bodies. This milk is great on cereals and in smoothies.

4 cups Brazil nuts (soaked 8 hours) 1 Tbsp. vanilla 1 pinch sea salt
6 cups mineralized water 1 tsp. cinnamon

Rinse Brazil nuts well and drain. Blend 2 cups nuts and 3 cups water in a high-powered blender. Repeat. Save nut meat for other recipes, stored in a refrigerated airtight container. (Use within 24 hours.) Blend nut milk with vanilla, cinnamon, and sea salt.

Plan ahead by soaking nuts 8 hours. The whole process of milking them should take about 20 minutes beginning to end!

Superfood Smoothies

Smoothies are great meals if they're made with the right ingredients. They're also a terrific source of fiber, since they're blended as whole fruits and vegetables. Our smoothies at 118 are all packed with superfoods as a way of getting extra vitamins and minerals in every delicious sip.

— MERRY MONKEY SMOOTHIE —

"The Monkey" smoothie is the number one favorite at 118 and is packed with protein. There are even variations on it now, such as the Chocolate Mint Monkey, Green Monkey, and Mango Monkey. This recipe is also great for kids—it tastes just like a milk shake!

1 peeled banana	1 Tbsp. agave nectar	1 cup ice
2 Tbsp. almond butter or raw almonds	1 tsp. cinnamon	¼ cup Almond Milk (page 17)

Blend all ingredients well in a high-powered blender. For a Chocolate Mint Monkey, add 2 Tbsp. cacao powder and 8 large mint leaves. For a Green Monkey, add 2 leaves kale. For a Mango Monkey, add ½ ripe organic mango.

— AVOCADO WHIP SMOOTHIE —

The first time I (Jenny) went to Hawaii, I had an avocado smoothie—I thought it was the strangest thing. *Oh well, I'll try it,* I thought. One sip and I was hooked!

1 ripe Hass avocado	2 Tbsp. hemp seeds	½ cup ice
1 cup chopped pineapple	1 Tbsp. agave nectar or raw honey	½ cup water
1 ripe mango	½ peeled banana	

Blend all ingredients well in high-powered blender. Garnish with a pinch of hemp seeds and a hibiscus flower for color.

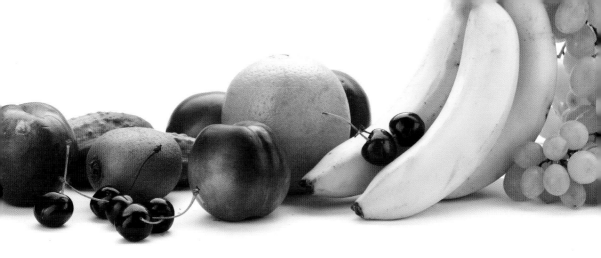

— PEACHES-AND-CREAM SMOOTHIE —

This smoothie is like dessert in a cup—an amazing blend of fruit, spices, and cream!

2 ripe peaches
1 ripe peeled banana
1 tsp. vanilla extract or 2 vanilla beans
½ cup Almond Milk (page 17)

2 Tbsp. almond butter
2 Tbsp. agave nectar
1 pinch Himalayan salt

½ cup ice
1 tsp. cinnamon

Blend all ingredients well in a high-powered blender and pour into a large chilled glass. Sprinkle with vanilla beans, and garnish with a cinnamon stick.

— FABULOUS FIG SMOOTHIE —

When figs are in season, there's nothing better than this smoothie! A little-known fact about this fruit is that it's high in protein. Enjoy this smoothie seasonally when figs are readily available at your local farmers' market!

1 ripe peeled banana
6 ripe mission figs
1 tsp. vanilla extract or 1 vanilla bean

1 tsp. maca-root powder
1 tsp. cinnamon
½ cup hemp milk

½ cup ice
1 tsp. hemp protein

Blend all ingredients well in a high-powered blender. Chop some additional fresh figs to float on the top, or place on the side of the glass for garnish.

— SWEET STRAWBERRY SMOOTHIE —

Strawberries are high in vitamins and minerals, and the coconut in this smoothie contains essential fatty acids. This smoothie makes the perfect meal for any time of the day.

> 8 strawberries, rinsed and de-stemmed
> 1 peeled banana
> 1 young Thai coconut (water and flesh)
> 2 Tbsp. hemp seeds
> 1 Tbsp. agave nectar

Blend all ingredients in a high-powered blender. Pour into chilled hurricane glasses, and garnish with strawberry slices.

— SUPERGREEN SMOOTHIE —

A great way to get your greens without having a salad is to blend them into a smoothie. You're also getting enough beneficial fiber to last you throughout the day. The best part? You can't taste the green!

> 1 ripe peeled banana
> 1 ripe mango, cut and peeled
> 2 leaves kale or 1 cup spinach
> 1 Tbsp. SuperGreens or spirulina
>
> 1 Tbsp. maca-root powder
> 1 tsp. agave nectar
> 1 cup young Thai coconut water
> ½ cup ice

Blend all ingredients well in a high-powered blender. Pour into a glass, and garnish with slices of banana or a fruit skewer to enjoy as a meal or appetizer! Or take in a travel mug on the road, especially in the morning.

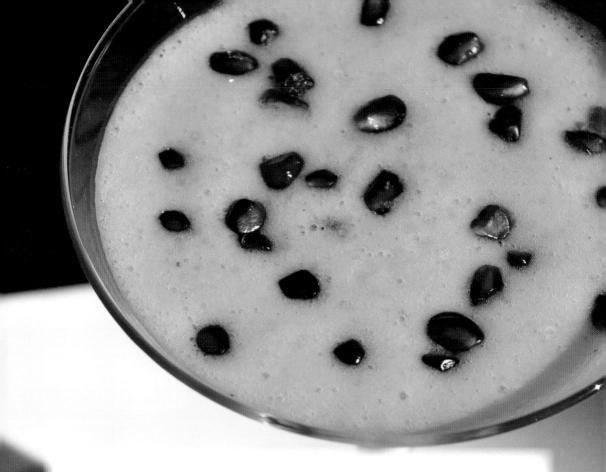

— POMEGRANATE-PASSION SMOOTHIE —

Pomegranates are extremely high in antioxidants; and this drink combines that high-intensity superfood with the sweet, mellow mango. The result is a mild smoothie that is hydrating, invigorating, and satisfying for every cell of your body.

1 cup pomegranate seeds or ½ cup pomegranate juice
1 young Thai coconut (water and flesh)
1 tsp. bee pollen (optional, or substitute with maca-root or mesquite powder)

1 whole mango, cut and peeled
1 Tbsp. agave nectar
1 cup ice

Blend all ingredients well in a high-powered blender, and enjoy. This recipe is great with a little buckwheat granola and banana sprinkled on top as well.

— BALANCE SMOOTHIE —

Balance can sometimes be elusive in a stressful environment and in daily life, with a growing list of things to do. This recipe provides balance internally, in the hopes that you may then see that balance reflected in your outer world. This smoothie calls for superfoods, some of which are balancing Chinese herbs.

½ mango
½ peeled banana (freeze prior to use)
½ cup ice
1 package Juvo (can be replaced with 1 tsp. SuperGreens or E$_3$Live,
  1 tsp. reishi mushroom, 2 Tbsp. tocotrienols, and 1 Tbsp. maca-root powder)

½ cup nut milk (see page 17 for recipes)
½ cup spinach
2 Tbsp. hemp seeds

Blend all ingredients in a high-powered blender, and then pour into a glass. Garnish with hemp seeds and a banana spear.

— DANCING-RAINBOW SMOOTHIE —

This smoothie recipe is just plain fun. It's about light, happy energy that you can add to your day for that extra kick to get you through!

1 ripe peeled banana
2 leaves kale
½ cup hemp milk
1 ripe mango or 1 cup cut pineapple

4 Tbsp. raw cacao nibs
1 Tbsp. maca-root powder
1 tsp. vanilla extract or 1 vanilla bean
1 Tbsp. matcha green-tea powder

Blend all ingredients in a high-powered blender. Garnish with fresh fruit rolled in hemp seeds. Enjoy!

— Chocolate Supreme Smoothie —

Raw cacao is high in magnesium and other creativity enhancers. This superfood smoothie is great for unlocking your mind's potential to create, and it also provides a naturally stimulating energy. The most important thing about this recipe is that it's balanced by rich green foods.

1 ripe peeled banana or avocado	2 Tbsp. hemp seeds
1 young Thai coconut (water and flesh)	2 Tbsp. agave nectar
2 Tbsp. raw cacao nibs or powder	1 tsp. cinnamon
1 Tbsp. maca-root powder	1 Tbsp. SuperGreens or spirulina
1 tsp. vanilla extract or 1 whole vanilla bean	½ cup ice

Blend all ingredients well in a high-powered blender. Pour into a glass lined in Chocolate Sauce (page 134) and serve, or sprinkle with fresh cinnamon and garnish with a cinnamon stick!

— Zen Energy Smoothie —

This drink promotes sustained energy throughout the day. Maca root, with its full chain of amino acids, is powerfully adapted in the body, which means that it provides energy. Matcha is unrefined, unroasted green tea, used in Asian cultures for years as an anti-aging drink. The two in combination will leave you feeling awake—yet very Zen.

1 ripe peeled banana	2 leaves kale or ½ cup spinach
1 cup Almond Milk (page 17)	2 Tbsp. agave nectar
1 Tbsp. almond butter	1 tsp. vanilla flavor or 1 vanilla bean
1 Tbsp. maca-root powder	1 tsp. cinnamon
1 Tbsp. matcha green-tea powder	½ cup ice

Blend all ingredients well in a high-powered blender. Transfer to a frosty mug or travel mug, and enjoy the energy all day long!

Chapter Two

Super Salads

Super salads are a great foundation for a vibrant living-foods diet. We enjoy at least one a day.

What makes a salad super? The ingredients, of course! When you transition to a living-foods diet, one of the most important keys to success is consuming at least 70 percent fresh fruits and vegetables. Salads are a great way to do this!

At the 118 restaurant, all of our salads are tossed with rich, flavorful dressings; a wide variety of colorful fruits and vegetables; organic fresh greens; and of course . . . love! Please enjoy these salads as entrées on their own, or share with family and friends. Salads are a great way to get a meal going and a fabulous opportunity to try fresh, in-season vegetables from your local farmers' market.

Shopping for Greens

Greens are best when sourced locally and organic, providing protein, chlorophyll, vitamins, and minerals. Check your local farmers' market for the freshest selection. Pick a different type of green you haven't tried before each time you shop. A few that might shake up your salad include:

- **Organic mixed baby greens:** This blend can be referred to as mesclun, field, or spring mix, depending on the greens included.

- **Spinach:** Popeye's power food, spinach is rich in iron, protein, and lutein for healthy connective tissue, muscular development, and overall nutrition.

- **Mustard greens:** These have a spicy flavor that goes well with avocado and cucumber, and they're particularly good for detoxification.

- **Lacinato and other kale varieties:** Kale is a great choice, as it is high in chlorophyll, vitamins C and K, and calcium, among other nutrients.

- **Arugula:** This herb has a strong flavor and is great mixed into other, lighter greens, like baby romaine.

- **Collard greens:** Collards are a nice option for wraps, as the leaves are large enough to roll. They're also great marinated with garlic-infused olive oil.

- **Rainbow chard:** Chard grows in a rainbow of colors, with the brighter hues being the sweetest, and provides a good deal of fiber.

- **Sprouts:** Try sunflower, broccoli, and onion sprouts and sprouted legumes. Flavorful and full of protein, sprouts are a bioavailable source of vitamins and minerals, for instant energy!

- **Fresh leafy herbs:** Basil, cilantro, and mint are nice additions to your salad and are perfect for use as a garnish.

- **Romaine hearts:** Romaine is typically light and crispy, and can be found in heirloom varieties with bright purple heads.

- **Napa cabbage:** This cabbage is great shredded, or since the leaves are nice and crisp, they can be used as taco shells and more.

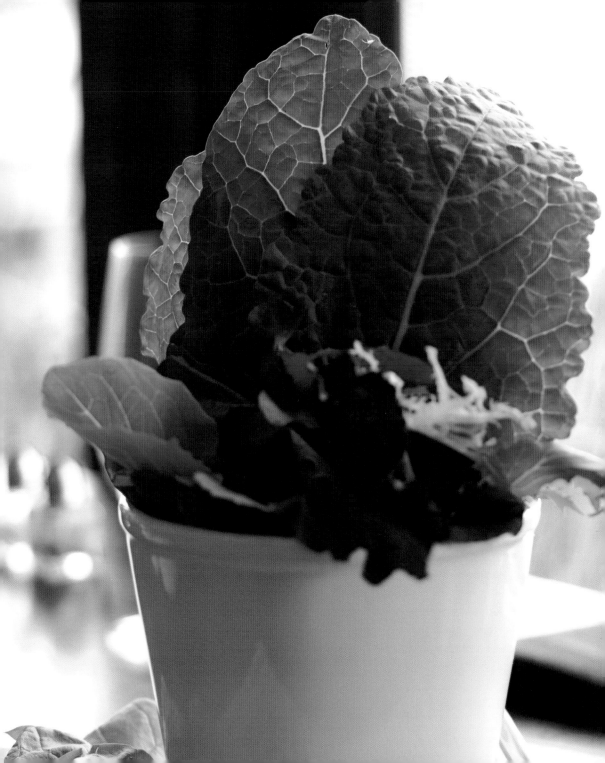

Salads

In the recipes that follow, ingredients marked with an asterisk (*) require advance preparation.

— SUMMER BERRY SALAD —

Fresh blackberries and strawberries, organic mixed greens, and a decadent dressing make this salad a sweet surprise and a customer favorite at 118. Berries are at their peak in the summer months and can be enjoyed right off the vine.

SALAD:
8 cups fresh salad mix

1 pint blackberries

1 ripe Reed avocado

2 cups strawberries

SALAD DRESSING:
¼ cup strawberries

1 cup pine nuts (soaked 4–6 hours)

¼ cup lemon juice

½ cup young Thai coconut water

1 Tbsp. agave nectar

1 tsp. Himalayan salt

Dressing preparation:
Rinse and drain pine nuts. Blend all ingredients in a high-powered blender, and chill until ready for use (lasts up to 7 days in the refrigerator).

Makes 1½ cups dressing.

Salad preparation:
Begin by thinly slicing all strawberries. In a glass or bamboo mixing bowl, toss salad, blackberries (save a few for garnish), avocado, and 1 cup salad dressing. For best results, toss well by hand, making sure the berries break up into the mixture. In an inverted 4-inch ring mold with removable top, layer thinly sliced strawberries, then salad mixture about halfway, and another layer of strawberries. Finish by filling in the second half of the mold with salad, and compress firmly. Invert mold and gently release salad by pushing top plate through. Garnish with fresh blackberries and a dollop of dressing.

Makes 4 servings.

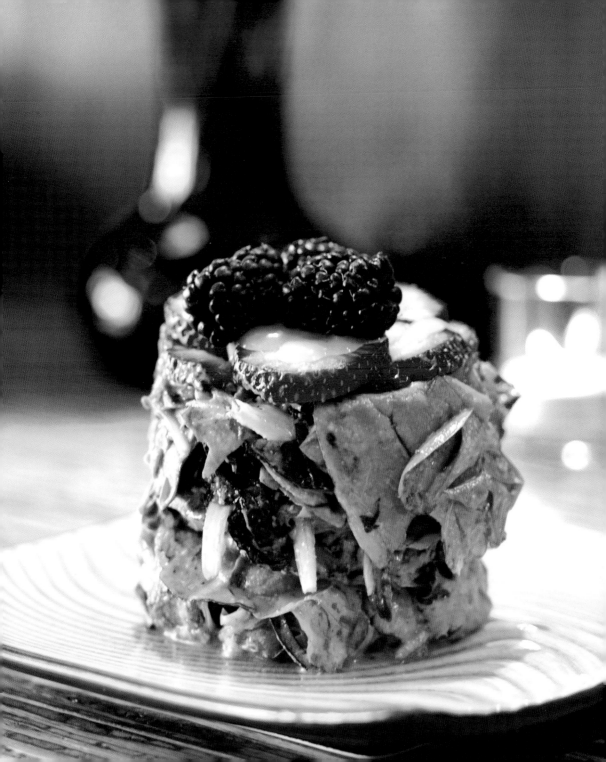

— CINNAMON FIG SALAD —

Figs are an excellent source of protein. Share this salad with family and friends as an excellent party dish. It's optimally enjoyed when figs are in season but can also be made with soaked dried figs.

SALAD:

6 cups baby romaine leaves

2 cups Caesar Dressing (page 90)

1½ cups Cinnamon Figs* (see below for preparation)

8 Tahini Cheese Figs* (see facing page for preparation)

In a large mixing bowl, combine Cinnamon Figs, romaine leaves, and dressing to coat greens. Toss well. Present on a flat plate and top with 2 Tahini Cheese Figs per serving. Garnish with fresh fig halves and a drizzle of dressing around plate.

Makes 4 servings.

Recipe suggestion: When using reconstituted figs, be sure to soak them at least 3 hours. If you'd like, you can use the soak water in the dressing, replacing the apple juice.

— CINNAMON FIGS —

2 cups fresh mission figs

4 Tbsp. agave nectar

1 tsp. cold-pressed extra-virgin olive oil

2 tsp. cinnamon

1 pinch Himalayan salt

2 tsp. vanilla flavor or 1 whole vanilla bean

Begin by carefully cutting stems off figs. Slice figs length wise in ¼-inch strips. Blend remaining ingredients in a blender. In a small mixing bowl, pour glaze over figs (save 8 slices for use in Tahini Cheese Figs—see facing page). Place figs on dehydrator tray covered in nonstick drying sheet, and dehydrate at 115° for 4 hours. Carefully pull from sheet and set aside for use in salad. Best if used warm.

— Tahini Cheese Figs —

8 fig slices (saved from Cinnamon Figs recipe)
4 Tbsp. Tahini Cheese (page 81)

Place fig slices onto nonstick drying sheet, and spoon ½ Tbsp. Tahini Cheese over each slice. Dehydrate at 115° for 4 hours while drying Cinnamon Figs.

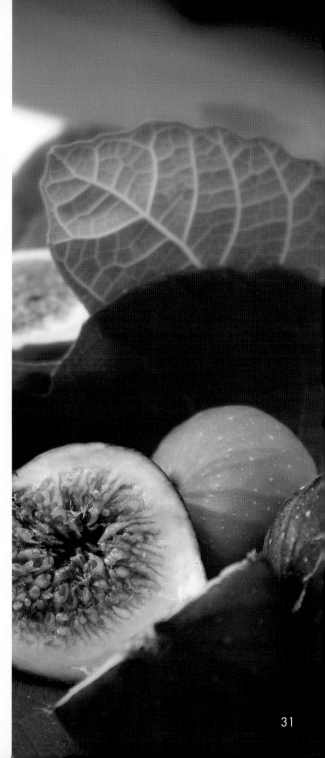

— TACO SALAD —

¡Olé! This salad will tap-dance on your taste buds with a delicious cilantro-chipotle dressing and a wonderful combination of Latin veggies. The *pepitas*, or pumpkin seeds, are very high in magnesium and are a great source of essential fatty acids. Enjoy as a starter course or as an entrée.

SALAD:

8 cups red romaine leaves
1 cup corn (about 1 ear)
3 cups marinated Latin Vegetables (page 44)
½ cup Spicy Pepitas, for garnish*
  (see facing page for preparation)

1 large Hass avocado
2 carrots, shredded
¼ cup Rojo Salsa, for garnish (page 100)

SALAD DRESSING:

4 oz. cold-pressed extra-virgin olive oil
4 oz. lemon juice
4 oz. young Thai coconut water
1 cup pine nuts (soaked 4–6 hours)
1 Roma tomato
½ red bell pepper

1 tsp. agave nectar
1 dried chipotle pepper
½ cup de-stemmed cilantro
1 clove garlic
1 Tbsp. dark chili powder
1 tsp. Himalayan salt

Dressing preparation:

Rinse and drain pine nuts. Blend all ingredients well in high-powered blender and use immediately or refrigerate for up to 7 days.

Makes 2 cups dressing.

Salad preparation:

Place organic greens, vegetables, and avocado in a large mixing bowl. Toss in dressing until well coated. Top with pepitas and serve. *Fun serving suggestion:* place the salad in avocado skins as an appetizer.

Makes 4 servings.

— SPICY PEPITAS —

2 cups raw pepitas (soaked 2 hours)   1 Tbsp. chili powder
1/8 cup cold-pressed extra-virgin olive oil   1 Tbsp. agave nectar
1 Roma tomato   1 Tbsp. dulse flakes
1 red bell pepper   1 tsp. coarse sea salt
1 clove garlic   1 tsp. cayenne pepper

Rinse and drain pepitas. Blend all ingredients (except pepitas) in a high-powered blender, and pour over soaked pepitas in a midsize mixing bowl. Spread out over nonstick drying sheet, and place in dehydrator at 115° for 12 hours. Rotate tray and stir mixture about 6 hours into drying.

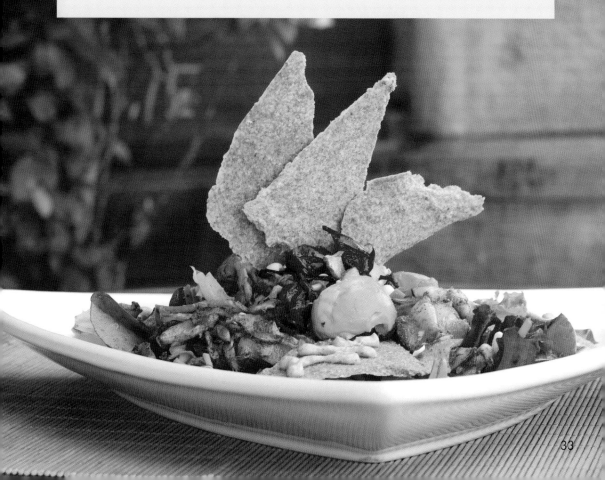

— Caesar Salad —

Our Caesar Salad at 118° is a top seller! This original twist on the classic Caesar provides a high density of nutrient value, including B vitamins and iron.

6 cups baby romaine lettuce
1 large Hass avocado, diced
3 Tbsp. capers
1/8 cup dulse, pulled into pieces
1/8 cup Basil Cheese, for garnish*
    (see page 36 for preparation)
2 cups Caesar Dressing (page 90)

Combine greens, avocado, dulse, and capers in large mixing bowl. Lightly toss with dressing until well coated. Place on serving plates or in wide-rimmed bowls. Garnish with Basil Cheese and enjoy as a starter or entrée!

Makes 4 appetizer-sized portions.

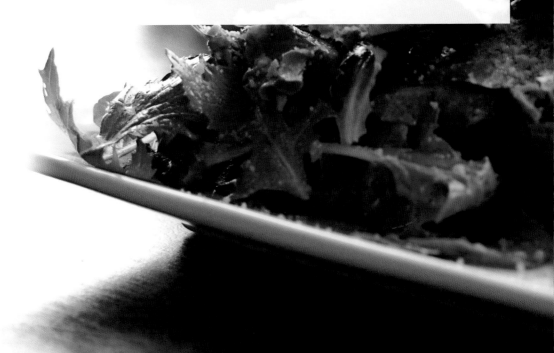

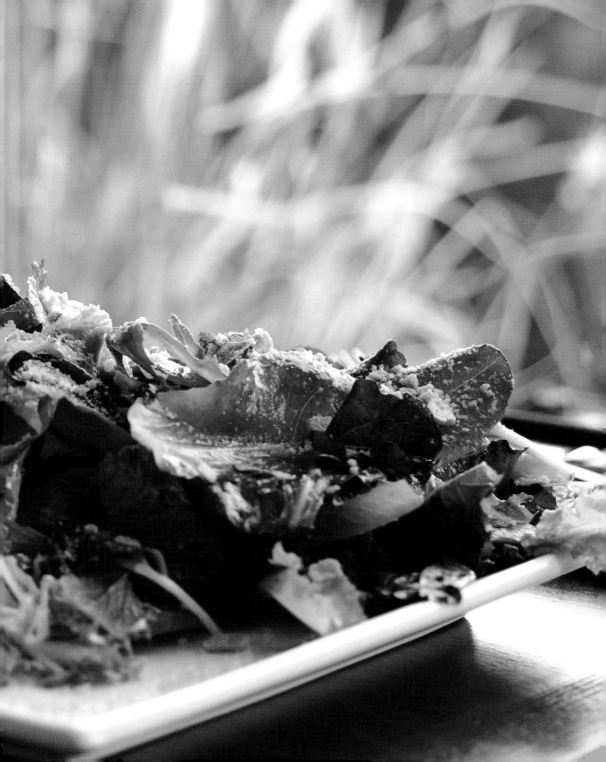

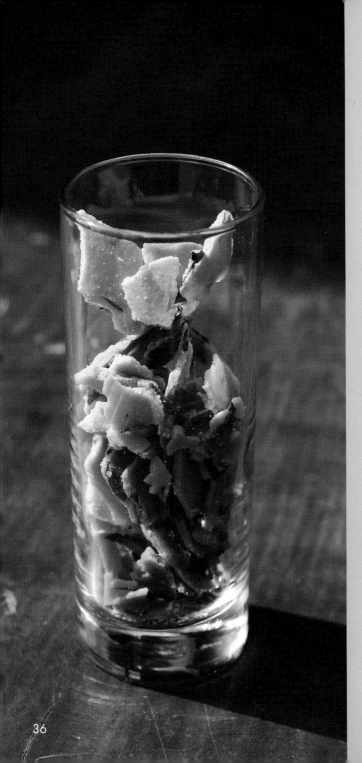

— BASIL CHEESE —

4 cups pine nuts
2 cups fresh basil, chopped fine
$\frac{1}{8}$ cup lemon juice
1 cup water
4 cloves garlic
1 tsp. Himalayan salt
1 Roma tomato

Blend all ingredients (except basil) in a high-powered blender until well mixed. Pour into midsize mixing bowl, and fold in chopped basil. Mix well. Spread over 2 dehydrating trays $\frac{1}{8}$-inch thick. Dehydrate at 110° for 12 hours. Break up into desired-size pieces, or crumble into fine cheese topping. The cheese saves 14 days in an airtight container and is great on soups and salads and over pizzas!

Makes 2 trays.

—Gorgeous Green Salad—

This salad is packed with chlorophyll, trace minerals, protein, iron, and B vitamins. It's a great one to add to your diet throughout the week as a staple of vibrant living.

Salad:
½ head kale
2 cups chopped spinach or mixed greens
1 cup chopped mustard greens
½ cup walnuts
1 large Hass avocado
½ cup sun-dried black olives
½ large hothouse cucumber, chopped into ¼-inch-thick rounds
½ cup dried dulse

Salad dressing:
4 oz. flaxseed oil
4 oz. lemon juice
1 clove garlic
1 Tbsp. dulse flakes
1 tsp. sea salt
1 dash cayenne
1 tsp. miso paste (optional)

Dressing preparation:
Blend all ingredients in a high-powered blender and refrigerate until use. This dressing will keep 10 days in the refrigerator.
Makes 1 cup dressing.

Salad preparation:
Finely chop kale and mustard greens and place in a large mixing bowl with ½ cup dressing. Carefully massage dressing into greens until well broken down. Blend in remaining greens, olives, walnuts, avocado, dulse, and chopped cucumber. Toss all ingredients well and enjoy straight from the bowl if you like!
Makes 1 entrée-sized serving.

— SHIITAKE SALAD —

Shiitake mushrooms have been used medicinally in Asian cultures for years to enhance health. In our salad, they offer a vital source of rich minerals and protein. Enoki mushrooms are another key ingredient that stimulates the immune system and is antiviral.

This salad is quick and easy to make and pairs fabulously with our Asian Infusion pasta, Thai Spring Rolls, and Curry Cones.

SALAD:

6 cups herb-salad mixed greens
1 cup enoki mushrooms, de-stemmed and rinsed
6 large shiitake mushrooms, de-stemmed and rinsed
$\frac{1}{8}$ cup fresh stemmed cilantro

1 hothouse cucumber, julienned
$\frac{1}{4}$ cup chopped green onions
2 large Hass avocados, diced

SALAD DRESSING:

8 oz. cold-pressed extra-virgin olive oil
4 oz. fresh lemon juice
1 Tbsp. miso paste
1 tsp. stone-ground mustard

1 clove garlic
1 tsp. agave nectar
1 dash cayenne pepper
1 inch green onion

Dressing preparation:

Blend well and chill until ready for use. This dressing will keep 10 days in the refrigerator.

Makes 2 cups.

Salad preparation:

Slice shiitake mushrooms lengthwise into $\frac{1}{4}$-inch-thick pieces. Add 2 Tbsp. salad dressing, and toss well so that all mushrooms are well coated. Add mixed greens, avocado, cilantro, green onions, and cucumber. Toss well. For serving, split into equal portions and top with enoki mushrooms; garnish with additional cilantro and green onions for an extra-spicy bite!

Makes 4 servings.

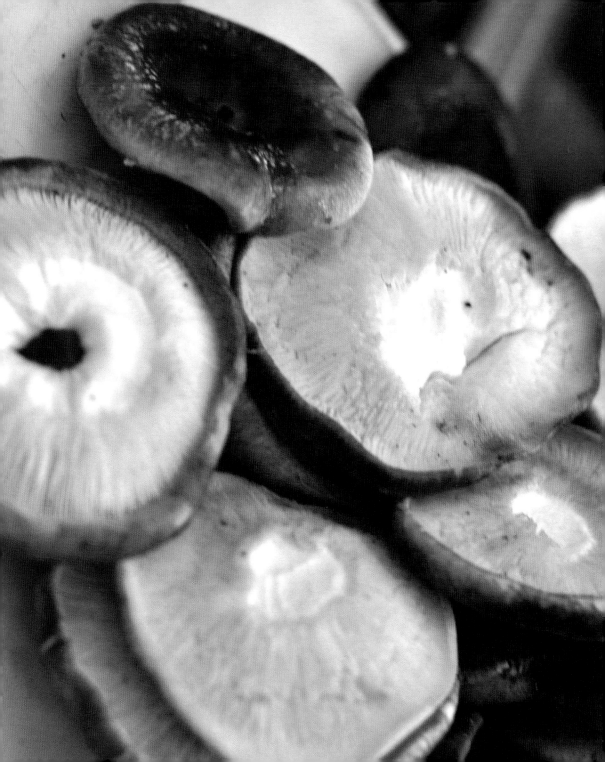

— SWEET PESTO SALAD —

This sweet and creamy pesto salad is packed with flavor and is sure to delight any palate. It goes perfectly with Italian meals and makes an excellent crispy lunch on its own. The olives provide a nice source of essential fatty acids to help with digestion.

SALAD:

8 cups mixed greens, spinach, or crispy romaine hearts

1 cup grape tomatoes, halved

½ cup Crispy Tomatoes, for garnish* (see facing page for preparation)

4 Tbsp. capers

½ cup olives

SALAD DRESSING:

2 cups cold-pressed extra-virgin olive oil

1 cup fresh basil

½ cup pistachios (soaked 4 hours)

2 Tbsp. agave nectar

3 cloves garlic

¼ cup lemon juice

1 tsp. coarse sea salt

Dressing preparation:

Rinse and drain pistachios. First blend olive oil, garlic, and basil to form green emulsion; then add soaked pistachios, agave, lemon, and sea salt. Blend well until thick and creamy. Use immediately or refrigerate for up to 10 days, keeping in mind that the oil will get thicker when cold—it may be a good idea to leave outside refrigerator for 15 minutes before using.

Makes 1½ cups dressing.

Salad preparation:

Combine organic greens, capers, grape-tomato halves, and olives in a large mixing bowl and coat well with dressing (about 1 cup) until thoroughly mixed. Pile high on serving plate and serve family-style, garnished with Crispy Tomatoes!

Makes 4 servings.

— CRISPY TOMATOES —

8 Roma tomatoes, rinsed
1/4 cup cold-pressed extra-virgin olive oil
3 Tbsp. agave nectar
1 clove garlic

1 dash cayenne pepper
1 tsp. coarse sea salt
2 Tbsp. dried Italian seasoning

Carefully slice Roma tomatoes into 1/4-inch-thick rounds by hand, or run through food processor on slicing blade. In blender, combine oil, agave, garlic, 1/2 tsp. sea salt, and pepper. Blend until well mixed. In a midsize mixing bowl, combine sliced Roma tomatoes and liquid mixture, and sprinkle in remaining sea salt. Toss with your hands to coat the tomatoes. Place well-coated tomatoes on nonstick drying sheet, and put into dehydrator set at 115° for 12 hours until very crispy. This garnish lasts up to 14 days in an airtight container once completely dried. Enjoy on salads, pizzas, and more!

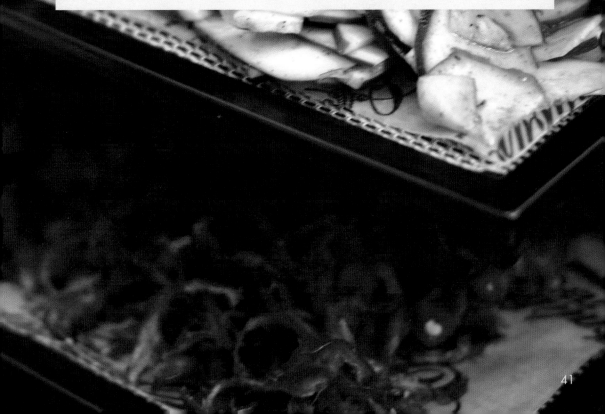

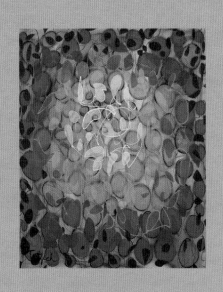

Chapter Three

Marinated Vegetables

Marinating is a quick and easy way to change the texture of vegetables and impart a richer flavor. In the winter, it's nice to enjoy them right out of the dehydrator in order to warm the body.

The basic technique of marinating vegetables is very simple and consists of four easy steps:

1. Pick a vegetable (squash, bell pepper, mushroom, onion, tomato, eggplant, and so on). Vegetables that are easiest to marinate are somewhat starchy and will soak up an oily marinade easily, like zucchini.

2. Prepare the vegetables by washing well and slicing thin, about $1/8$- to $1/4$-inch thickness.

3. Create a marinade. This can be as simple as blending 8 oz. of olive oil with 2 cloves of garlic for a quick garlic marinade. The following section includes some suggested recipes that are easy and fun to prepare. Remember that using dried spices is a great way to yield a variety of flavors!

4. Dehydrate. The goal here is to dehydrate the vegetables enough to soften the texture and cause them to soak up the marinade without losing their vital water content. To do this, you simply need to line a dehydrator tray with a nonstick drying sheet and layer the vegetables about $\frac{1}{2}$-inch thick across the tray.

Most vegetables will take about 2 hours to really reach an ideal texture and taste. The longer they're left in the dehydrator, the more intense the flavor of the marinade and the drier their texture.

Marinated Vegetables

Use the preceding section as a guide for vegetable marinades referenced throughout this book. Here are some of the more common mixtures used at 118:

— LATIN VEGETABLES —

2 medium squash (either zucchini or yellow squash)
2 red bell peppers
1 portobello mushroom
8 oz. cold-pressed extra-virgin olive oil

1 clove garlic
1 tsp. agave nectar
1 tsp. sea salt or Himalayan salt
2 Tbsp. dried chili powder

Thinly slice all vegetables. In a blender, combine oil and spices into a quick marinade by briefly blending. Pour over vegetables, and place on 2 dehydrator trays covered with nonstick sheets. Dehydrate at 110° for 2 hours.

Makes 4 cups.

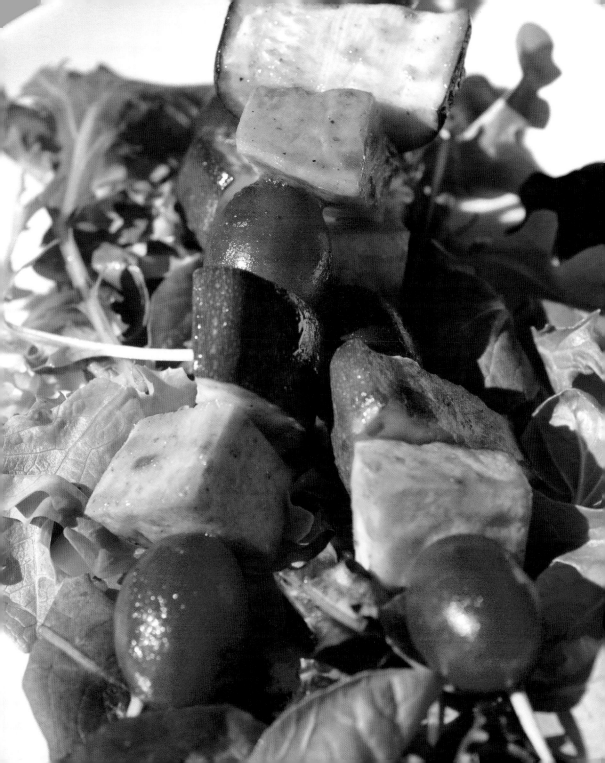

— ITALIAN VEGETABLES —

3 medium squash (either zucchini or yellow squash)
2 portobello mushrooms
8 oz. cold-pressed extra-virgin olive oil
2 Tbsp. dried Italian seasoning or ½ cup fresh basil
1 clove garlic
1 tsp. sea salt or Himalayan salt

Thinly slice all vegetables. In a blender, combine oil and spices into a quick marinade by briefly blending. Pour over vegetables, and place on 2 dehydrator trays covered with nonstick sheets. Dehydrate at 110° for 2 hours. Makes 4 cups.

— BBQ VEGETABLES —

2 medium squash (either zucchini or yellow squash)
3 red bell peppers
3 Roma tomatoes
½ large eggplant
1 portobello mushroom
8 oz. cold-pressed extra-virgin olive oil
2 Tbsp. dried chili powder
1 clove garlic
1 green onion (white portion only)
1 tsp. agave nectar
1 tsp. sea salt or Himalayan salt
1 dash cayenne pepper

Thinly slice all vegetables. In blender combine oil, 1 tomato, 1 red bell pepper, and spices into a quick marinade by briefly blending. Pour over remaining vegetables, and place on 2 dehydrator trays covered with nonstick sheets. Dehydrate at 110° for 2 hours. Makes 4 cups.

— Sweet Vegetables —

2 medium squash (either zucchini or yellow squash)
2 red bell peppers or 2 Roma tomatoes
1 ear bicolor corn
1 sweet brown onion
8 oz. cold-pressed extra-virgin olive oil

2 tsp. agave nectar
1 shallot
1 clove garlic
1 tsp. sea salt or Himalayan salt

Thinly slice all vegetables. In a blender, combine oil, shallot, and spices into a quick marinade by briefly blending. Pour over vegetables, and place on 2 dehydrator trays covered with nonstick sheets. Dehydrate at 110° for 2 hours. Makes 4 cups.

— Curry Vegetables —

2 medium squash (either zucchini or yellow squash)
2 shiitake mushrooms
1 yellow bell pepper
8 oz. cold-pressed extra-virgin olive oil

2 Tbsp. yellow curry powder
1 clove garlic
1 tsp. agave nectar
1 tsp. sea salt or Himalayan salt

Thinly slice all vegetables. In a blender, combine oil and spices into a quick marinade by briefly blending. Pour over vegetables, and place on 2 dehydrator trays covered with nonstick sheets. Dehydrate at 110° for 2 hours. Makes 4 cups.

— Spicy Spanish Squash —

2 zucchini or yellow squash, sliced thin
2 Tbsp. chili powder

1 tsp. cayenne pepper
1 tsp. sea salt

Combine ingredients in a medium-sized mixing bowl and toss until all squash is well coated. Spread out vegetables on 2 dehydrator trays covered in nonstick drying sheets, and dehydrate at 110° for 2 hours. Makes 2–3 cups.

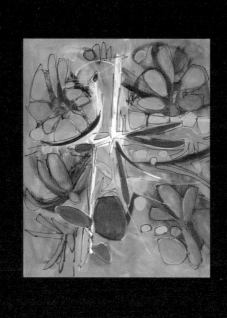

Chapter Four

Small Bites and Appetizers

Appetizers are perfect to enjoy with family and friends any time of the day and make great snacks to indulge in by yourself. Several of these work as a nice savory meal and are designed to be enjoyed tapas-style, with many small plates on a table at once.

These recipes are meant to tempt the taste buds of newcomers to living cuisine. All of the flavors and textures are easily enjoyed by a variety of palates, and presentation is a key component.

Carpaccios

Carpaccios are a lovely way to enjoy fresh vegetables without sacrificing flavor or texture. They make a very nice, light dish, especially in the spring and summer seasons. The two carpaccios in this section are universally enjoyed.

— EGGPLANT CARPACCIO —

1 large eggplant
2 cups cold-pressed extra-virgin olive oil
2 cloves garlic
1 Tbsp. aged balsamic vinegar
1 tsp. Himalayan salt
1 cup chopped basil

Prepare eggplant by slicing ½ inch off the top and bottom and discarding. Cut eggplant in half lengthwise, and then slice into ⅛-inch-thick pieces on a mandoline or by hand using a sharp chef's knife. Place in a medium-sized mixing bowl. In a blender, combine olive oil, garlic, and Himalayan salt and puree into garlic oil. Pour mixture over the top of eggplant and toss until well coated.

Place eggplant on dehydrator tray covered in a nonstick drying sheet, and dehydrate at 110° for 2 hours until soft and juicy. Lay out thin slices in a gently overlapping pattern, and drizzle with balsamic vinegar. Finish with chopped basil and enjoy!

Makes 6 appetizer servings.

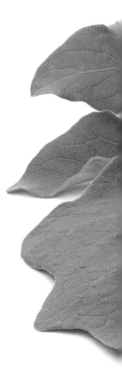

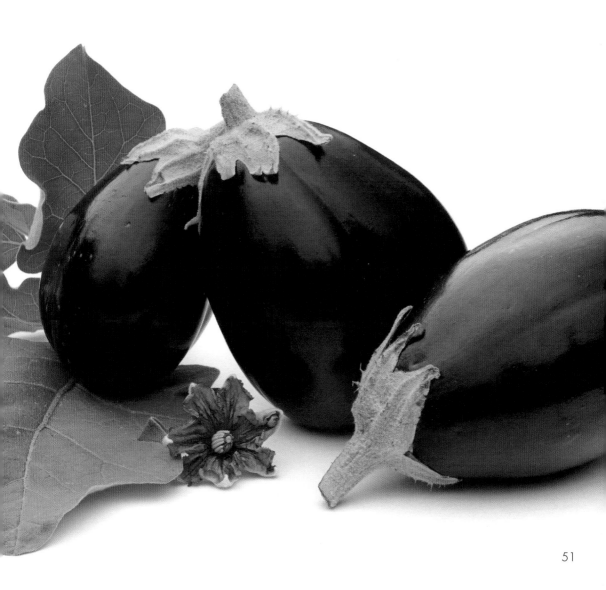

— ZUCCHINI-ASPARAGUS CARPACCIO
WITH BASIL CHEESE —

This recipe was inspired by a local organic farm in San Juan Capistrano, California, offering a beautiful community-supported agriculture (CSA) program, which means that consumers can buy bushels of various types of produce directly from the farmers on a weekly or biweekly basis. Thank you, South Coast Farms!

2 medium-sized zucchini
6 asparagus spears
$\frac{1}{4}$ cup capers
2 Roma tomatoes
$\frac{1}{4}$ cup cold-pressed extra-virgin olive oil
1 dash sea salt
Basil Cheese, for garnish (page 36)

Using a mandoline set at $\frac{1}{8}$ inch, thinly slice strips of zucchini. Cut Roma tomatoes into $\frac{1}{8}$-inch-thick rounds. Using a Y peeler, carefully peel asparagus strips. Pour olive oil and sea salt in a glass mixing bowl. Gently coat tomato and zucchini strips, and set aside for immediate use; then toss asparagus strips in remaining liquid.

Gently place tomatoes in one layer across bottom of serving plate. Layer with zucchini strips; then top with capers, asparagus mixture, and finally a sprinkling of Basil Cheese.

Makes 4 appetizer servings.

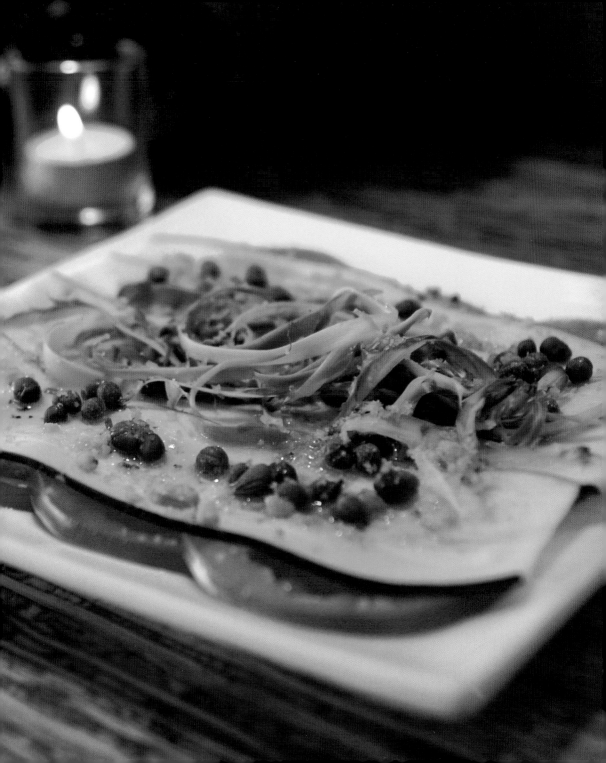

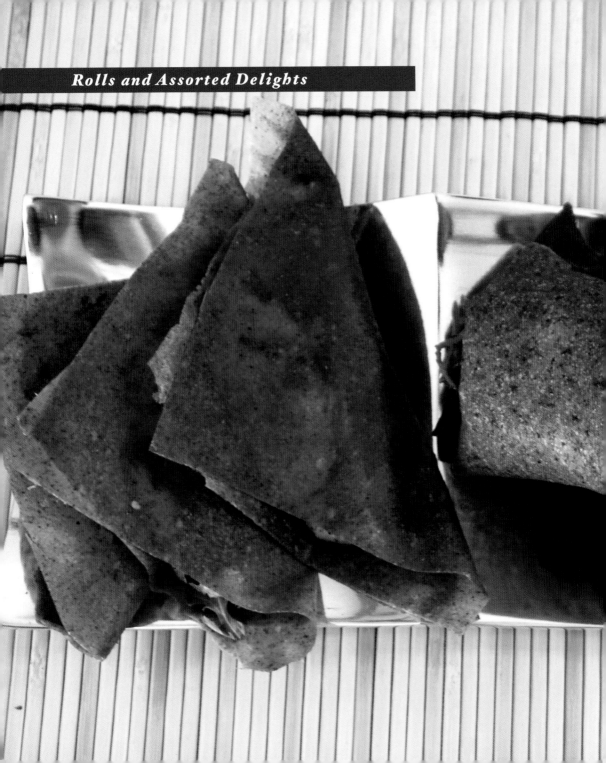

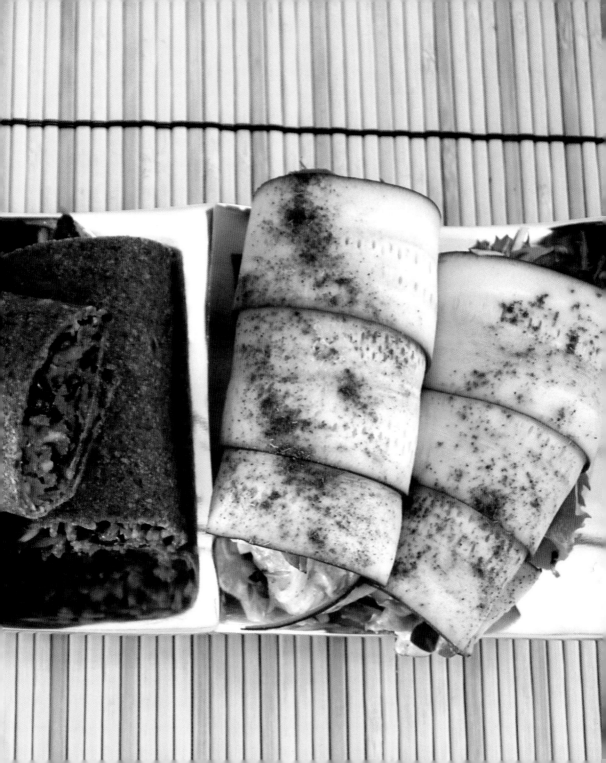

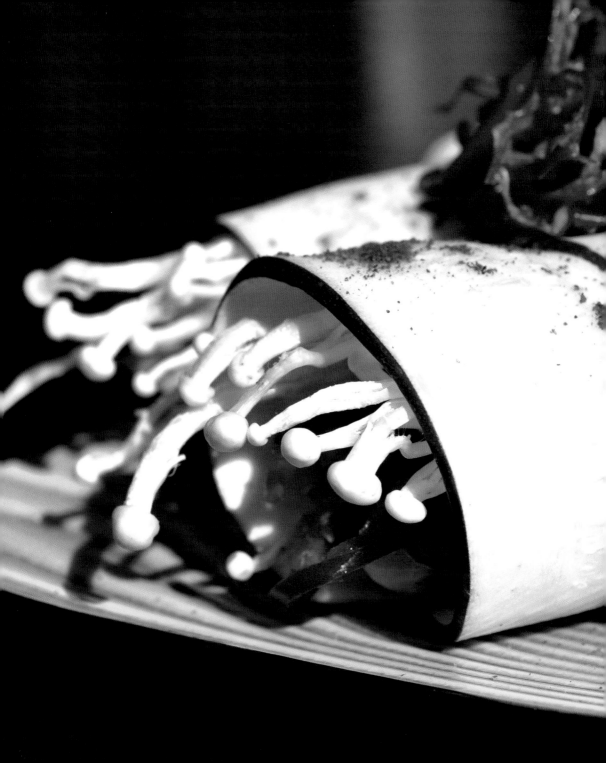

— NUMI ROLLS —

One morning in the warm summer months, I (Jenny) was in the kitchen yearning for a crisp and vibrant snack. These rolls evolved from that day's produce and have been a hit among my product line and in my store ever since. This light, fresh preparation takes 10 minutes or less to make.

ROLL:
2 zucchini

FILLING:
1 ripe Hass avocado (cut lengthwise into 8 slices per half)
1 red bell pepper (cut lengthwise very thin)
1½ cups shredded beets or carrots
1 Roma tomato (cut thin)
1 cup fresh spinach leaves
4 green onions
¼ cup Chipotle Cheese (page 83)

Prepare zucchini by slicing off and discarding both ends where previously attached to the vine. Slice zucchini lengthwise on a mandoline set at ⅛ inch. On a cutting board, line up 3 pieces of zucchini next to one another, overlapping by ¼ inch. In the middle of each set of zucchini, layer vegetables across, beginning with the spinach, then shredded carrots or beets, Roma tomato, red bell pepper, avocado, and green onions. Finally, add 3 Tbsp. Chipotle Cheese per roll. Gently roll up zucchini tightly around vegetables. Sprinkle with dried Italian spices or cayenne pepper (depending on your preference) and enjoy.

Makes 6 appetizer servings.

— STUFFED MUSHROOMS —

Yum! This recipe can be created with either cremini or shiitake mushrooms, since both are equally delicious. Mushrooms provide a unique source of protein and offer a great texture that's especially enjoyable for beginners to living-foods cuisine.

MUSHROOMS:
16 shiitake or cremini mushrooms, cleaned and de-stemmed
4 Tbsp. cold-pressed extra-virgin olive oil

FILLING:
2 cups pistachios (soaked 4 hours)
1 cup cold-pressed extra-virgin olive oil
1 cup basil
5 cloves garlic
1 tsp. Himalayan salt

TOPPING:
½ cup grape tomatoes, chopped into 4 round slices each

Begin by placing mushrooms in a medium-sized mixing bowl with 4 Tbsp. olive oil, and lightly toss until well coated. Rinse and drain pistachios. In a high-powered blender, combine olive oil, basil, garlic, and salt. Puree until dark green in color. Add pistachios and blend to a creamy texture.

Fill each mushroom cap with filling mixture, and place on dehydrator tray covered in nonstick drying sheet. Top with grape-tomato slices, and dehydrate at 105° for 4 hours. The longer you leave the mushrooms in the dehydrator, the softer they become, and the stronger and more intense their flavor, as well as that of the garlic. These have a long shelf life in the refrigerator—just dehydrate them to revive their flavor and serve them warm!

Makes 8 appetizer servings.

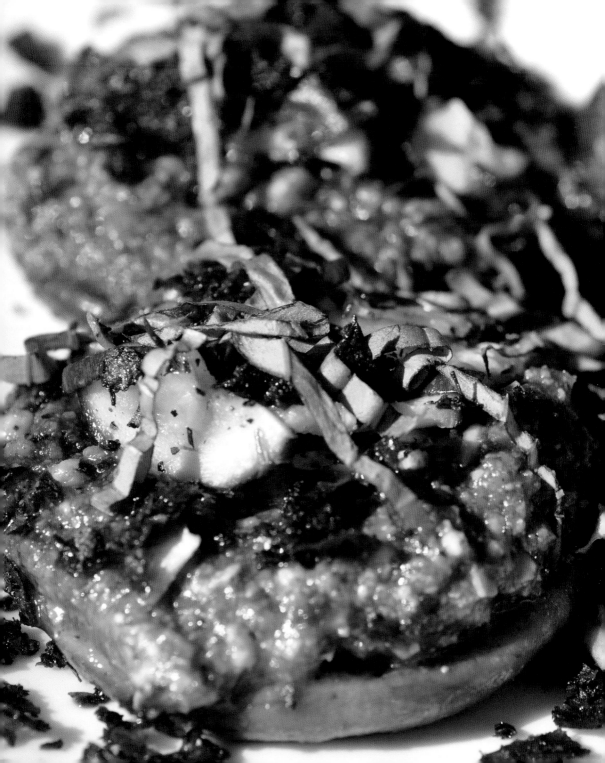

— SHIITAKE SUSHI ROLLS —

This is a quick and easy recipe for energy any time of the day, yet delicate enough for your next dinner party. These sushi rolls can be served on a fresh nori sheet or Thai Coconut Wrap (page 94), depending on your preference.

PIGNOLIA RICE:
2 cups pine nuts (soaked 2 hours)   2 tsp. lemon juice
2 cloves garlic   1 Tbsp. miso
1 tsp. Himalayan salt

VEGETABLE FILLING:
2 cucumbers, julienned   4 green onions, chopped
1 cup shredded carrots   2 ripe Hass avocados, sliced
2 cups thinly sliced shiitake mushrooms   1 cup Miso Dressing (page 87)
1 cup clover sprouts

GARNISH:
1 cup Sweet Cheese (page 82)   Juice of 1 lemon

Rinse and drain pignolias (pine nuts). Begin by combining pignolia-rice ingredients in a food processor with S blade in place. Process until sticky rice-like mixture forms, remove from processor, and set aside. (Mixture will save for up to 5 days in refrigerator.)

On a large cutting board, lay out 4 pressed raw nori sheets or 4 quarters of Thai Coconut Wrap. Next, press rice onto wraps from the bottom to the middle in 1/8-inch-thick layer. In a small mixing bowl, blend shiitake mushrooms with Miso Dressing until dressing is well absorbed. Beginning with mushrooms, layer vegetables until all wraps have a thin layer of each one. Carefully roll wraps around vegetables. Finish by gently wetting your fingers and moving them along the top of each wrap to cause it to stick to itself. Cut at a diagonal for a nice handheld sushi roll.

For a garnish, gently whisk together Sweet Cheese and lemon juice and place in a demitasse cup for dipping. *Optional:* add 1 tsp. ginger juice and 1 tsp. cayenne to the mixture for a nice kick.

Makes 8 appetizer servings.

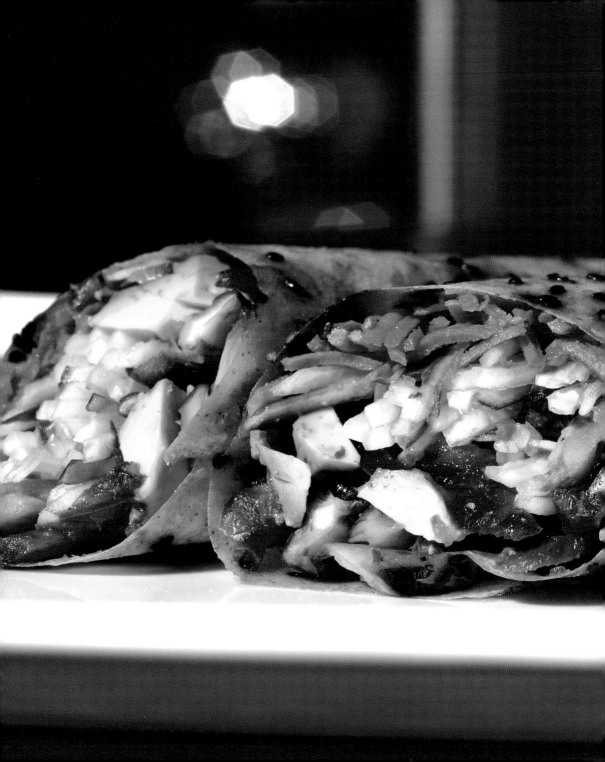

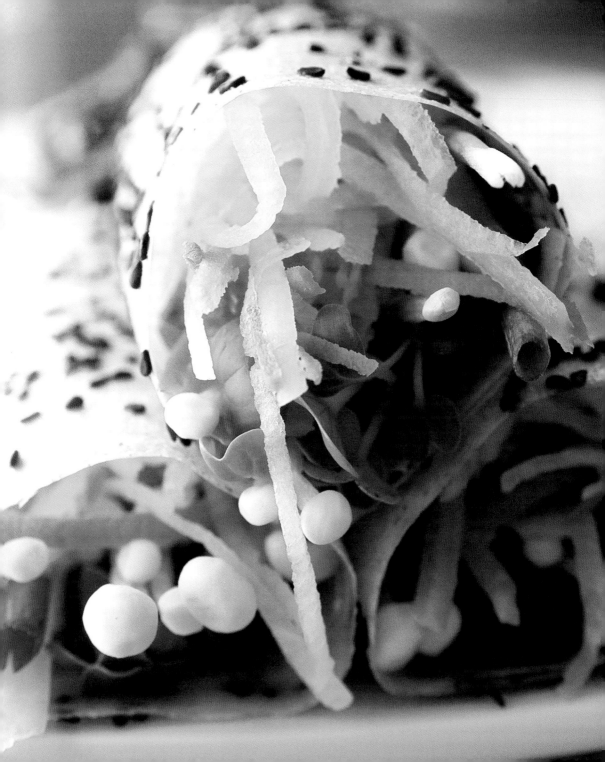

— Thai Spring Rolls —

These spring rolls are a number one bestseller on the menu at 118 any time of the day. The sweetness of the wrap combines with the delicate crunch of fresh vegetables for a memorable roll. Serve these to friends and family year-round!

Wrap:
Use 1 tray Thai Coconut Wrap (page 94)

Filling:
1 cup shredded carrots
2 thinly sliced red bell peppers
1 cup shredded green papaya
2 ripe Hass avocados
1 package enoki mushrooms
1 cucumber, julienned
1 zucchini, julienned

Sauce:
1 cup Avocado-Lime Sauce (page 91), Sweet Cheese (page 82), or Red Bell Pepper Puree (page 87)

Begin by cutting 1 tray of Thai Coconut Wraps in half lengthwise. Further cut each half into 3 equal sections, totaling 6 pieces. Lay out all pieces on a large cutting board, and layer fresh vegetables inside wrap about 2 inches from bottom. Roll tightly and stack rolls next to each other on a platter. Serve with sauce to garnish.

Makes 6 appetizer servings.

— PESTO ROLLS —

This roll is served sushi-style and requires very little work besides the advance preparation of the wrap and marinated vegetables.

WRAP:
Use 1 tray basil Coconut Wrap (page 94)

FILLING:
2 zucchini, julienned
1 cup shredded carrots
2 thinly sliced red bell peppers
1 cup Pistachio Pesto (page 86)
4 Tbsp. Sun-Dried-Tomato Marinara (page 89)

GARNISH:
1 cup marinated portobello mushrooms
4 Tbsp. Sun-Dried-Tomato Marinara (page 89)

Begin by cutting basil Coconut Wrap in half lengthwise. Carefully spread ½ cup Pistachio Pesto on each wrap, stopping ½ inch from the top. Layer vegetables lengthwise halfway through each wrap, beginning with the carrots, then squash (spread 2 Tbsp. marinara evenly over top), and finally red bell peppers. Gently roll wrap to form one long 1½-inch-thick roll.

Cut rolls in half and further cut each half into 4 equal pieces. Set pieces on their sides next to one another, and top with marinara and portobello mushrooms before serving.

Serve with chopsticks for a fun presentation . . . these rolls can also be eaten as a finger food!

Makes 8 appetizer servings.

— Curry Cones —

This recipe is a flavorful delight, especially as the summer turns to fall. Enjoy these handheld wraps with friends while sitting around a fire talking about what dreams may come to fruition during the year!

Wrap:
Use 1 tray curry Coconut Wrap (page 94)

Filling:
1 cup shredded carrots
1 cup shredded beets
1 cup Spicy Spanish Squash (page 47)
1 cup marinated red bell peppers
1 cup freshly chopped spinach
1 cup Pistachio Pesto (use pine-nut version of recipe (page 86)

Dipping sauce:
1 cup Red Bell Pepper Puree (optional) (page 87)

Begin by cutting curry Coconut Wrap in half lengthwise. Cut halves into 3 sections each. In a medium-sized mixing bowl, combine filling ingredients and toss until well mixed. Place equal portions of mixture into each wrap lengthwise, and gently roll into a cone shape. Garnish with little soufflé cups filled with Red Bell Pepper Puree for dipping.

Makes 6 appetizer servings.

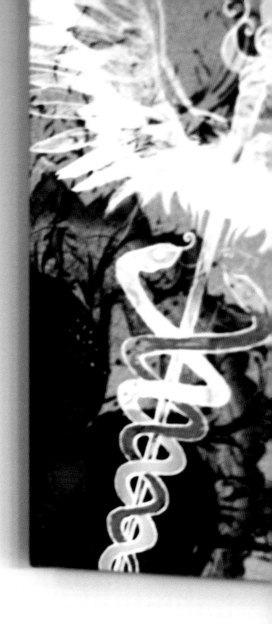

— EMPANADAS —

An Argentine specialty, these empanadas evoke a sense of warmth, comfort, and home-style love. The filling suggested below is the house blend at 118, but you might want to mix up the vegetables based on what's freshest at your local farmers' market. (We also encourage you to dance in the kitchen when preparing these special treats . . . but, of course, it's all up to you!)

DOUGH:

2 cups sprouted Kamut® grain or wheat berries (sprouted 3–5 days)   1 Tbsp. chili powder
½ cup ground golden flaxseed   1 tsp. sea salt

FILLING:

2 cups Almond Cheese (page 82)   1 cup ground golden flaxseed (for rolling)
1 cup Latin Vegetables (page 44)   2 ears corn (cut off cob)

GARNISH:

2 cups Avocado-Lime Sauce (page 91)

Begin by placing Kamut grain in a food processor with S blade in place. Process until well broken down (meaning that there are no full grains left). Add flaxseed, chili powder, and sea salt, processing until dough ball begins to form. Remove dough and set aside. On a medium-sized cutting board, spread ground golden flaxseed to coat board.

Scoop out 2-inch balls of dough onto cutting board. Roll out into 4-inch oval-shaped pieces with nonstick rolling pin. Fill each empanada with 3 Tbsp. Almond Cheese and 3 Tbsp. vegetables. Fold empanadas over and indent edges. Place on dehydrator tray, and dehydrate at 110° for 5 hours or until dry to the touch. Enjoy warm! Garnish with Avocado-Lime Sauce on top, or on the side for dipping.

Makes 8 appetizer servings.

— Quinoa Cakes —

Quinoa is an ancient grain that's high in protein and has no gluten. This ingredient is easy to sprout and enjoy in its most vibrant form: *alive!*

Cakes:
  2 stalks celery
  1 large red beet
  2 cups sprouted quinoa (sprouted 8 hours)
  1 cup pine nuts (soaked 4–6 hours)
  ¼ cup fresh or reconstituted, soaked figs
  1 red bell pepper
  Juice of 1 lemon
  2 tsp. chili powder
  1 Roma tomato
  1 tsp. Himalayan salt

Garnish:
  1 cup Sweet Cheese (page 82)
  1 cup marinated red bell peppers

Rinse and drain figs, quinoa, and pine nuts. Juice celery and beet, and combine both the juice and pulp in a food processor with S blade in place. Add pine nuts, figs, red bell pepper, lemon, chili powder, tomato, and Himalayan salt. Process into puree. Add quinoa and process into thick grainy mixture. Using a 2-inch food scoop, scoop mixture into ball shapes on nonstick-drying-sheet-lined dehydrator tray, about 2 inches apart. Gently press each ball down into cake-like shape about ½-inch thick.

Dehydrate at 110° for 8–10 hours until soft but not overly crispy. Serve on plates garnished with Sweet Cheese and marinated red bell peppers for a colorful appetizer.

Makes 8 servings.

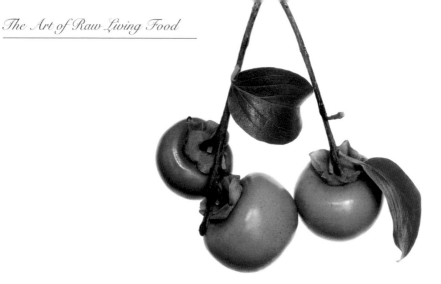

— **PERSIMMONS AND SAVORY CHEESE** —

A seasonal favorite, these sweet and savory treats are best enjoyed during the fall months and can be served fresh or lightly warmed in the dehydrator.

4 Fuyu persimmons (soft to the touch)
1 pomegranate
2 cups Tahini Cheese (page 81)

4 Tbsp. agave nectar
1 tsp. cinnamon

Begin by cutting each persimmon through the middle section, removing and discarding the top and bottom first, and then cut into 4 equal slices. Lay slices out evenly on cutting board. With an offset spatula, gently spread a thin layer of Tahini Cheese ⅛-inch thick across the top. (If you'd like to serve the persimmons warm, place in dehydrator at 110° for 45 minutes.)

Open pomegranate, remove seeds, and sprinkle them over persimmons. Garnish with agave nectar and a sprinkling of cinnamon.

Makes 4 appetizer servings.

— DEVILED TOMATOES —

Tomatoes with flair! These tasty treats can delight your dinner-party guests and are quick and easy to make. If you don't have a dehydrator, the tomatoes can be prepared the day before and left to sit and soak up flavor. They'll save for up to 3 days—a great snack to have around the house!

TOMATOES:

8 Roma tomatoes (the seeds and inside pulp will be used for the filling, see below)

FILLING:

1 cup tahini
1 cup lemon juice
2 red bell peppers
4 cloves garlic

2 Tbsp. agave nectar
2 tsp. chili powder
1 green onion (small white part only)

Begin by slicing Roma tomatoes in half lengthwise, and remove inside pulp and seeds with a coring tool for use in filling. Gently pat dry each tomato to remove excess juice. In a high-powered blender, combine red bell pepper, tomato filling, lemon juice, agave, garlic, green onion, and chili powder. Blend well. Add tahini and finish blending into thick paste. Spoon paste into center of Roma tomatoes, and line them up on dehydrator tray. Dehydrate at 110° for 4 hours until filling is set and tomatoes are soft and juicy. Serve warm.

Makes 8 appetizer servings.

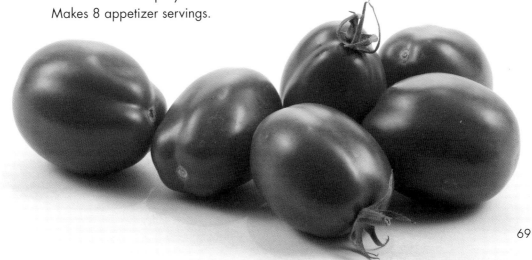

— New Mexico Nachos—

This rich and decadent plate of nachos is enough to make children—and adults—ooh and aah with enjoyment. Serve these on a large platter at your next get-together, or break them up into small portions for your own pleasure.

Chips:
16 Corn Chips (page 99)

Topping:
1 cup Chipotle Cheese (page 83)
1 cup Green Guacamole (page 101)
1 cup Sweet Cheese (page 82)
1 cup Rojo Salsa (page 100)
1 cup Spicy Spanish Squash (page 47)
1 cup marinated red bell peppers
2 bicolor corn, cut off cob
¼ cup nopales (cactus), diced
1 cup shredded carrots

Begin by layering 8 Corn Chips in a circular pattern on a serving platter.
Follow with carrots, guacamole, marinated squash, and Chipotle Cheese.
Add another layer of 8 chips and layer with red bell peppers, corn,
cactus, Sweet Cheese, and then salsa.
Makes 4 appetizer servings.

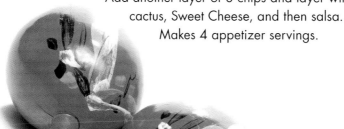

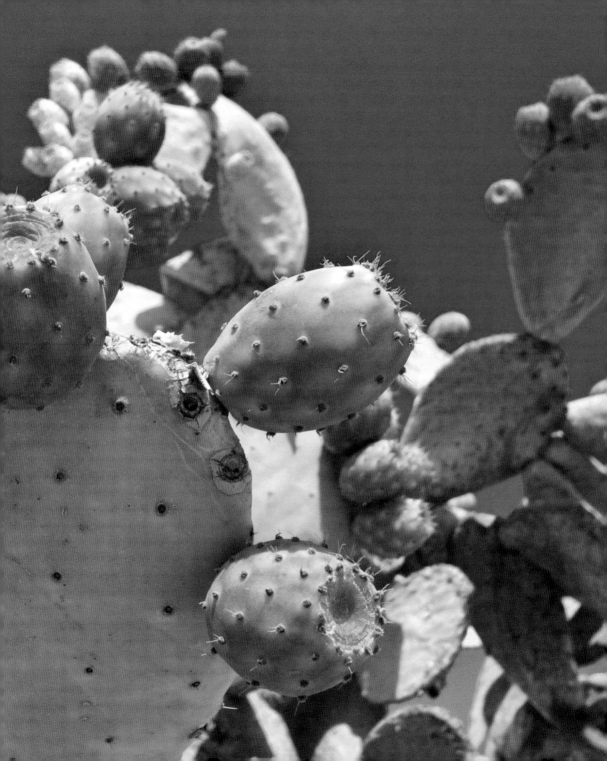

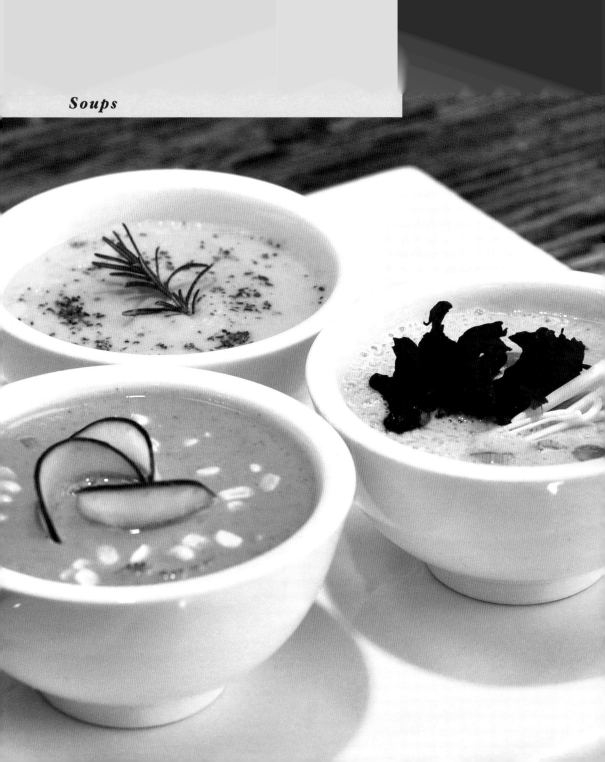

— SHIITAKE MISO SOUP —

This is a hearty miso soup, full of rich flavor!

SOUP:
6 shiitake mushrooms
½ cup Sweet Cheese (page 82)
2 cloves garlic
2 Tbsp. miso paste
1 tsp. sea salt
1 dash cayenne pepper
4 cups hot water

GARNISH:
½ cup dulse
10 enoki mushrooms (⅛ cup fresh de-stemmed cilantro can be substituted)
1 cup sliced shiitake mushrooms
1 green onion, chopped

Blend all soup ingredients in a high-powered blender until frothy and creamy. Pour into 4 bowls and garnish each with dulse, mushrooms, and a sprinkling of green onions.

Makes 4 appetizer servings.

— BUTTERNUT-SQUASH SOUP —

This is a wonderfully warming soup in the winter season! Enjoy it as a starter or a meal, garnished with Decadent Butternut Chips!

SOUP:

1 large butternut squash, diced (approx. 2½ cups)
¼ cup cold-pressed extra-virgin olive oil
¼ cup pine nuts
1 sprig fresh rosemary
½ Roma tomato
1 clove garlic
2 Tbsp. agave nectar
2 cups warm (110°) water
1 tsp. sea salt

DECADENT BUTTERNUT CHIPS:

1 cup butternut squash, diced
½ Roma tomato
2 tsp. dried Italian seasoning
1 clove garlic

¼ cup pine nuts
Juice of ½ lemon
1 tsp. sea salt

Preparation of chips:

Blend all ingredients in a high-powered blender. Spoon 2-inch rounds onto dehydrator tray covered in nonstick drying sheet. Dehydrate at 110° for 8–12 hours (will be crispy when finished).

Makes 25 chips.

Soup preparation:

Blend all the soup ingredients in a high-powered blender until well combined. Enjoy fresh from the blender with Decadent Butternut Chips, or save in the refrigerator for up to 5 days. *Helpful hint:* To warm, place soup in dehydrator at 115° for 20 minutes or lightly warm on stove for a brief period, testing temperature with thermometer or by touch (should be like bathwater).

Makes 4 appetizer servings.

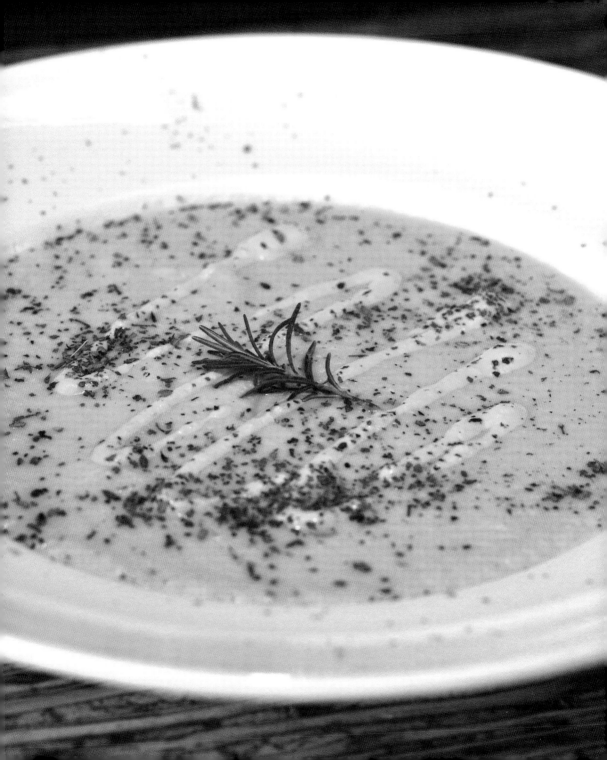

— TORTILLA SOUP —

A spicy companion to any Spanish meal and a great way to stay warm in the winter, our tortilla soup is rich and creamy and is beautifully garnished with fresh vegetables, avocado, and chips!

SOUP:
4 Roma tomatoes
1 cup pine nuts
1 red bell pepper
1 chipotle pepper
2 cloves garlic
2 Tbsp. chili powder
2 Tbsp. cold-pressed extra-virgin olive oil
Juice of 1 lemon
1 tsp. sea salt
2 cups hot water

GARNISH:
2 cups Spicy Spanish Squash (page 47)
2 ripe avocados, diced
8 Corn Chips (page 99)

Blend all soup ingredients in a high-powered blender until rich and creamy. Pour into small bowls for serving, and garnish each with squash and diced avocado. Top with 2 chips each.

Makes 4 appetizer servings.

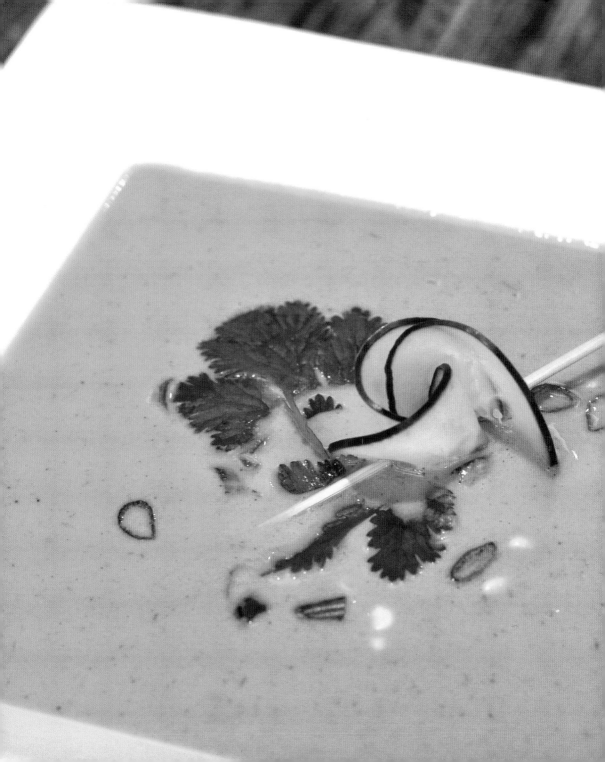

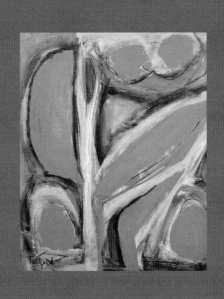

Chapter Five

Sauces, Spreads, Breads, and Crackers

Most of the recipes in this chapter can be made and saved for enjoyment throughout the week. They're cross-referenced in many other sections of the book and are found here with substitution options and instructions for storage. It's a good idea to prepare a few sauces, spreads, and snacks to enjoy without fuss on a weekly basis.

Many of these recipes call for a high-powered blender. We suggest a Vita-Mix brand blender (available at **www .shop118degrees.com**) with a plunging apparatus. These high-powered appliances can easily blend nuts, seeds, and thick pâtés that are challenging for normal blenders.

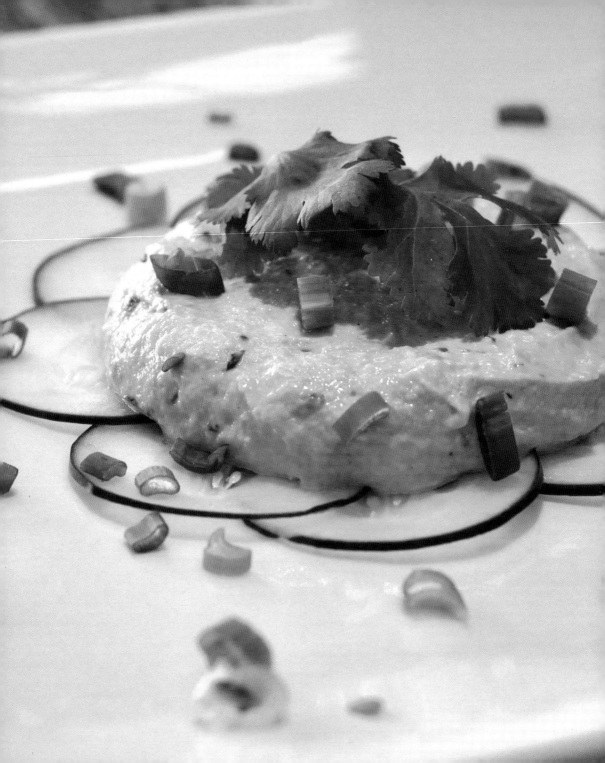

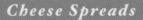

Cheese Spreads

— TAHINI CHEESE —

This is an all-time favorite at 118 and will become a delightful addiction if kept around in your kitchen. Tahini is high in calcium, which makes it a great part of your daily diet. This recipe can be made in advance and will keep for up to 10 days in the refrigerator.

16 oz. raw ground-sesame tahini
2 cups lemon juice
4 cloves garlic
¼ cup de-stemmed cilantro
⅛ cup chopped green onions
1 tsp. Himalayan salt

Begin by placing lemon juice, garlic, cilantro, green onions, and salt in food processor, and process until lightly mixed. Pour in the tahini from the top of processor while it's still running, and keep it on briefly just until the mixture turns a shade of white and becomes thick. Overprocessing will cause the cheese to become green and bitter, so if you're uncertain, use the "pulse" feature to make sure the mixture is well combined but doesn't become a puree.

Makes 2 cups Tahini Cheese.

— ALMOND CHEESE —

This naturally alkaline-forming cheese is flavorful and saves for up to 5 days in the refrigerator.

2 cups almonds (soaked 8 hours)
4 Tbsp. cold-pressed extra-virgin olive oil
2 Roma tomatoes
Juice of 1 lemon

2 cloves garlic
2 tsp. Himalayan salt
2 tsp. chili powder
1½ cups water

Rinse and drain almonds. In a high-powered blender, combine all ingredients and blend well. *Helpful tip:* add all liquids, herbs, and vegetables to the blender first; then follow with nuts to aid in ease of blending. Makes 2 cups.

— SWEET CHEESE —

This cheese is an all-purpose recipe that can be used in many different types of dishes, from Asian to Spanish. It will save for up to 5 days in the refrigerator.

2 cups pine nuts
1½ cups young Thai coconut water
Juice of 1 lemon
1 Roma tomato

2 Tbsp. agave nectar
2 cloves garlic
1 tsp. sea salt

Blend all ingredients well in a high-powered blender until thick and creamy. *Helpful tip:* this recipe can be made with macadamia nuts by substituting them for the pine nuts and adding 2 Tbsp. olive oil. Makes 2 cups.

— CHIPOTLE CHEESE —

Unique to 118's menu, this flavorful, smoky cheese saves for up to 7 days in the refrigerator and makes a nice addition to any Spanish dish!

2 cups pine nuts
1½ cups water
Juice of 1 lemon
1 Roma tomato

1 large dried chipotle pepper
2 tsp. chili powder
2 cloves garlic
1 tsp. sea salt

In a high-powered blender, combine all ingredients and blend until rich and creamy. *Helpful tip:* if you'd like this even spicier, add 1 tsp. cayenne pepper and another ½ dried chipotle pepper. Makes 2 cups.

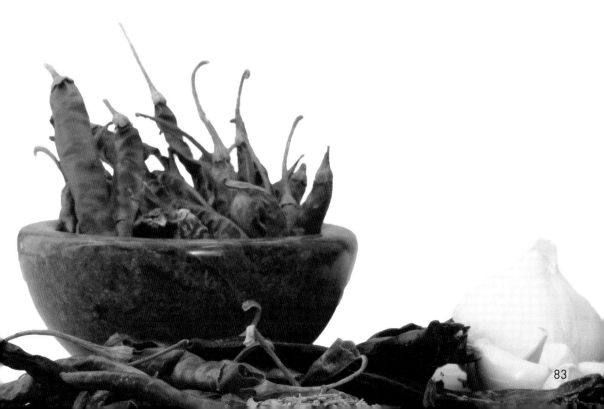

— MACADAMIA-SPINACH RICOTTA —

Ricotta cheese is naturally thick and creamy, making it an excellent spread for heartier dishes, and it's great on a crudités platter as well. This versatile ricotta is sure to please anyone's palate, and the leftovers can be dehydrated to form a savory topping for salads and soups. Inspired by a trip to Italy, this recipe has been a favorite for years.

4 cups macadamia nuts
1½ cups water
¼ cup cold-pressed extra-virgin olive oil
2 Roma tomatoes
4 cloves garlic
1 tsp. Celtic sea salt
Juice from 2 lemons
4 cups chopped spinach

Combine all ingredients (except spinach) in a high-powered blender. Begin blending on low, and gently turn to high as mixture begins to break down. Be sure to use a plunger or stop and scrape sides of blender to ensure that ingredients are well combined. Scrape out cheese and place in a medium-sized mixing bowl. Fold in chopped spinach and mix well using a spatula or wooden spoon. Refrigerate for up to 7 days, and dehydrate any leftover ricotta by spreading it thin over nonstick drying sheet and placing in dehydrator at 115° for 14 hours.

Makes 4 cups.

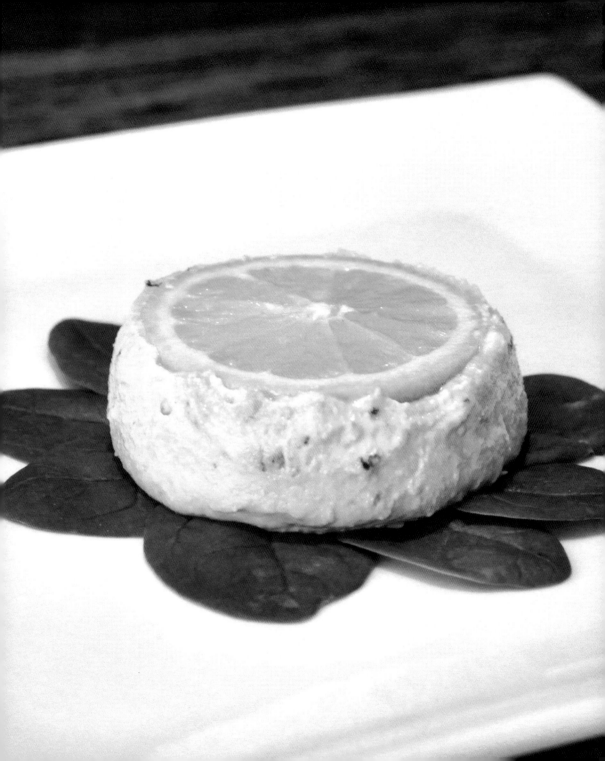

Sauces, Toppings, and Dressings

— PISTACHIO PESTO —

A rich and creamy pesto, this recipe is easy to make and saves for up to 14 days in the refrigerator.

8 oz. cold-pressed extra-virgin olive oil
2 cups fresh basil leaves
6 cloves garlic
2 cups pistachios (soaked 4 hours)

Rinse and drain pistachios. In a high-powered blender, combine olive oil, basil, and garlic. Blend well until a thick green oil forms. Add pistachios and blend until rich and creamy. *Helpful tip:* this recipe may be made with pine nuts as well.
Makes 2 cups.

— PINE-NUT SOUR CREAM —

This is a quick and easy recipe for sour cream that can be refrigerated for up to 7 days.

2 cups pine nuts
1½ cups water
Juice of 2 lemons
1 Roma tomato
2 Tbsp. agave nectar
3 cloves garlic
1 tsp. Himalayan salt

Blend all ingredients well in a high-powered blender until thick and creamy—great for use on sandwiches, to top soups, and even as a salad dressing!
Makes 2 cups.

— MISO DRESSING —

This is a light dressing blend that's easy to make and will save for up to 10 days in the refrigerator.

8 oz. cold-pressed extra-virgin olive oil
2 Tbsp. raw ground-sesame tahini
1 Tbsp. miso paste
2 cloves garlic
Juice of 2 lemons
8 cilantro leaves
1 green onion (small white bulb only)

Blend all ingredients well until mixture emulsifies. This works great as a marinade, as well as with mushrooms and eggplant.
Makes 1 cup.

— RED BELL PEPPER PUREE —

This is a simple vegetable puree that can be added to a variety of dishes. The sauce saves for up to 5 days in the refrigerator

6 red bell peppers
6 oz. cold-pressed extra-virgin olive oil
2 cloves garlic
1 tsp. sea salt

Blend all ingredients well in a high-powered blender until a thick puree forms. Some flavorful options include adding 1 tsp. cayenne pepper or 2 tsp. chili powder for a spicier blend, or 2 Tbsp. Italian herbs for a Mediterranean-style sauce.
Makes 1 cup.

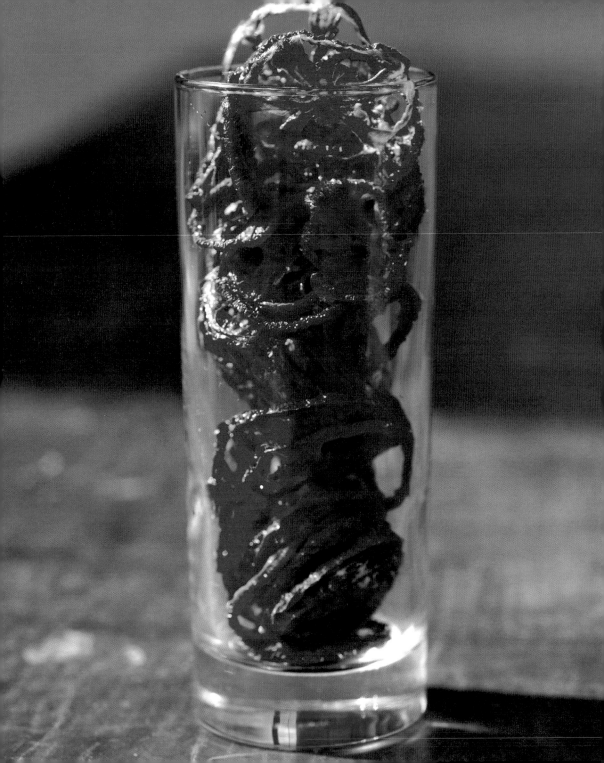

— SUN-DRIED-TOMATO MARINARA —

This rich marinara can be used with Italian dishes and can be stored up to 5 days in the refrigerator.

6 Roma tomatoes
6 oz. cold-pressed extra-virgin olive oil
4 Sun-Dried Tomato halves (recipe below)
2 Tbsp. agave nectar

5 leaves fresh basil
2 cloves garlic
2 Tbsp. dried Italian seasoning

Blend all ingredients well in a high-powered blender until rich and creamy. Makes 2 cups.

— SUN-DRIED TOMATOES —

A crispy, savory snack and garnish, this recipe makes excellent use of leftover tomato and is a great addition to salads and soups. Spice up the flavor and texture of any dish by adding some crumbles to the top before serving.

8 Roma tomatoes (or other tomatoes of your choice)
2 Tbsp. dried Italian seasoning
4 Tbsp. cold-pressed extra-virgin olive oil

2 Tbsp. agave nectar
1 tsp. sea salt

Begin by rinsing tomatoes well and cutting off the portion attached to the vine and discarding it. Then attach the slicing blade to a food processor and process all tomatoes into thin slices. (You can also cut them by hand into $1/8$-inch-thick slices). In a large mixing bowl, combine tomato slices, spices, olive oil, agave nectar, and sea salt. Toss until well coated. Carefully spread out on nonstick drying sheet, and place in dehydrator at 115° for 12 hours. To speed drying time, gently flip tomatoes over onto screen after 6 hours and continue drying the rest of the way. These tomatoes will keep for up to 2 months in an airtight container, but please make sure they are completely dry before storing in order to prevent fermentation.

Makes about 2 cups.

— GARLIC CRÈME SAUCE —

A light cream sauce that makes an excellent spread for sandwiches and a light filling for entrée dishes, this recipe pairs nicely with mushrooms, eggplant, and spinach. A garlic lover's delight!

2½ cups pine nuts (soaked 2 hours)
½ cup cold-pressed extra-virgin olive oil
Juice from 1 lemon or 1 tsp. apple-cider vinegar
2 large cloves garlic

1 tsp. Himalayan salt
1 Roma tomato
½ tsp. dried dill (optional)
4 Tbsp. capers (optional)

Rinse and drain pine nuts. Place pine nuts, tomato, lemon juice, garlic, and sea salt in a high-powered blender and begin blending. Add olive oil while blending in order to emulsify liquid until light and creamy. Add dill, if desired, and blend well. Toss in capers, if desired, and stir into mixture. Refrigerate for up to 10 days.
Makes 2½ cups.

— CAESAR DRESSING —

This is an amazingly delicious raw, vegan Caesar-style dressing that can be enjoyed on top of any salad or used as a marinade on vegetables or pasta dishes. It can be stored in the refrigerator for up to 7 days.

8 oz. cold-pressed extra-virgin olive oil
½ cup pine nuts
Juice of 2 lemons

2 cloves garlic
⅛ cup dulse leaves or flakes
1 tsp. Himalayan salt

Blend all ingredients well in a high-powered blender until rich and creamy dressing forms. Add a dash of cayenne pepper for an extra kick!
Makes 2 cups.

— AVOCADO-LIME SAUCE —

A unique blend of avocado, this sauce will keep in the refrigerator for up to 5 days . . . if you can make it last that long! It tastes great as a spread and a sauce and works well with Spanish and Continental cuisines.

2 ripe Hass avocados
4 oz. cold-pressed extra-virgin olive oil
1 cup young Thai coconut water
2 cloves garlic
Juice of 2 limes
1 tsp. Himalayan salt
1 tsp. agave nectar
1 dash cayenne pepper

Blend all ingredients well in a high-powered blender until a rich, creamy sauce forms. Enjoy!
Makes 2 cups.

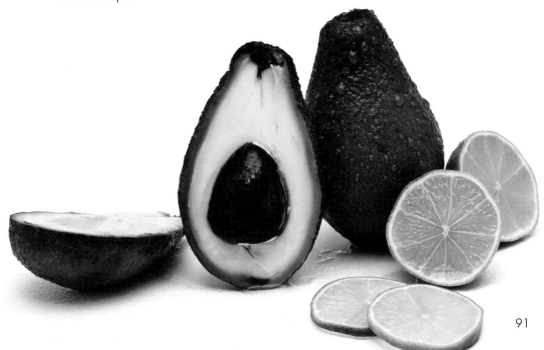

Breads are a great item to make on a biweekly basis and enjoy as pizza crusts, sandwich bases, and flatbreads. The variety at 118 is a soft, pliable flatbread that is lovingly prepared daily at the restaurant. The breads in this section are extremely high in protein and can be made with an array of sprouted grains. Keep in mind that they're very dense and a little goes a long way.

We use Kamut as our grain of choice. It's an ancient type made from an heirloom-variety seed that's low in gluten (although not completely gluten free). Wheat berries and rye could also be substituted in these recipes. For those with wheat sensitivities, rye is generally the best option. For people who are intolerant of gluten, we recommend sticking with the Almond Bread option (which uses flaxseed).

— OLIVE KAMUT BREAD —

The house bread at 118, this makes a great pizza crust, sandwich base, or snack with any of our spreads. Use it within 10 days.

4 cups sprouted Kamut grain (sprouted 3–5 days)	2 Tbsp. dried Italian seasoning
1½ cups sun-dried black olives	2 cloves garlic
4 Tbsp. cold-pressed extra-virgin olive oil	1 tsp. sea salt

Rinse and drain sprouted grain. In a food processor with an S blade attached, combine sprouted grain and olives and begin processing so that the grain begins to break down. As the mixture is processing, add garlic, Italian seasoning, and olive oil until a dough ball begins to form.

Gently press mixture about ¼-inch thick on 2 dehydrator trays covered in nonstick drying sheets. Dehydrate at 110° for 4 hours, flipping once halfway through.

— ALMOND BREAD —

Almond Bread is a great alternative to breads made with sprouted grains and is an excellent use of leftover pulp from milking almonds and juicing carrots. One of the most fulfilling parts of having a living-foods kitchen is that absolutely nothing has to go to waste. This is a great way to help preserve the planet and nourish your body at the same time. Living congruently with Mother Nature frees up space for more manifestation on every level.

4 cups almond pulp (from Almond Milk preparation—see page 17)
2 cups carrot pulp (saved from juicing)
1 cup ground golden flaxseed
2 Tbsp. cold-pressed extra-virgin olive oil

2 tsp. sea salt
2 cloves garlic
2 Tbsp. dried Italian seasoning

In a food processor with an S blade attached, combine all ingredients (except flaxseed) and process until a smooth mixture forms. Add ground golden flaxseed until a dough ball forms.

Press out onto covered dehydrator tray, and dehydrate at 110° for 8 hours, flipping once halfway through.

— ONION POPPY-SEED BREAD —

A very popular combination of flavors, this bread smells incredible as it begins to warm. Use it within 10 days of initial preparation.

4 cups sprouted rye or wheat berries (sprouted 3–5 days)
4 Tbsp. cold-pressed extra-virgin olive oil
4 Tbsp. poppy seeds

2 cloves garlic
½ sweet onion
1 tsp. sea salt

Rinse and drain sprouted grain. In a food processor with an S blade attached, combine sprouted grain and sweet onion and begin processing so that the grain starts to break down. As the mixture is processing, add poppy seeds, garlic, and olive oil until a dough ball forms.

Gently press mixture about ¼-inch thick on 2 dehydrator trays covered in nonstick drying sheets. Dehydrate at 110° for 4 hours, flipping once halfway through.

Wraps

— COCONUT WRAPS —

These wraps are a signature item at the 118 restaurant. They're designed with ease of digestion in mind and have been universally enjoyed. There are five signature varieties that are used throughout the book. These wraps can be made in advance, and they save for up to 30 days in the refrigerator.

4 cups young Thai coconut flesh   2 Tbsp. psyllium husk
2 cups water   Seasoning of choice*
1 tsp. agave nectar

Blend coconut, water, seasoning of choice, and agave in a high-powered blender. After thick creamy mixture forms, add psyllium husk and blend until mixture begins to congeal. Spread thin over 4 covered dehydrator trays, and dehydrate at 110° for 6 hours. Wrap will be dry to the touch yet still pliable.

*Saffron wrap:
  1 Roma tomato
  1 pinch Spanish saffron

*Spanish/tomato wrap:
  1 Roma tomato
  1 Tbsp. chili powder

*Basil wrap:
  1 cup finely chopped basil
  1 tsp. agave nectar

*Curry wrap:
  2 Tbsp. yellow curry powder
  1 tsp. agave nectar

*Thai wrap:
  1 tsp. agave nectar (sprinkle wrap with
    black sesame seeds after spreading)

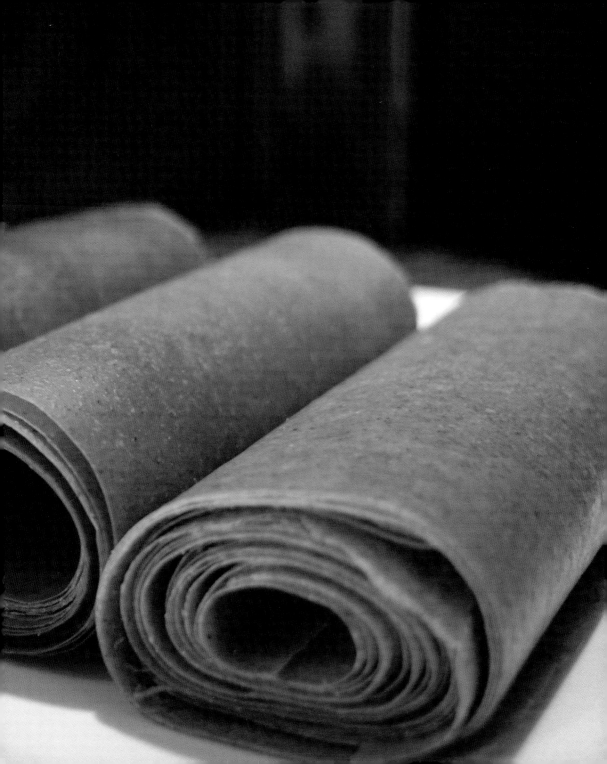

— Zucchini-Flax Wrap —

This is a very versatile wrap that can be used for up to 30 days after preparation. Be sure to store it in the refrigerator.

2 large zucchini
1½ cups ground golden flaxseed
2 Tbsp. dried Italian seasoning
2 cups water
1 clove garlic

Blend all ingredients well in a high-powered blender until thick and creamy. Flaxseed will cause the mixture to thicken, so be sure to transfer to covered dehydrator trays as quickly as possible. Spread thin in ⅛-inch-thick layer over 4 trays, and dehydrate at 110° for 4–6 hours. Make sure not to go over the time too long, as the mixture will eventually become crispy.

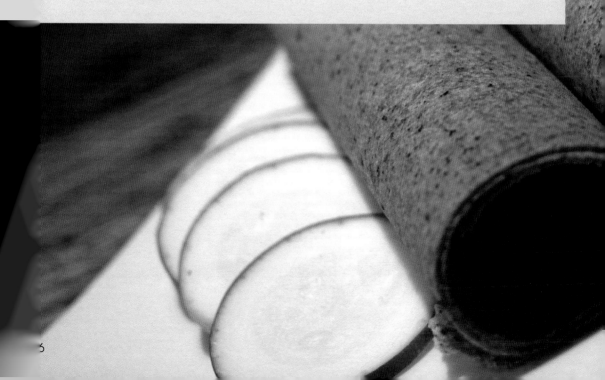

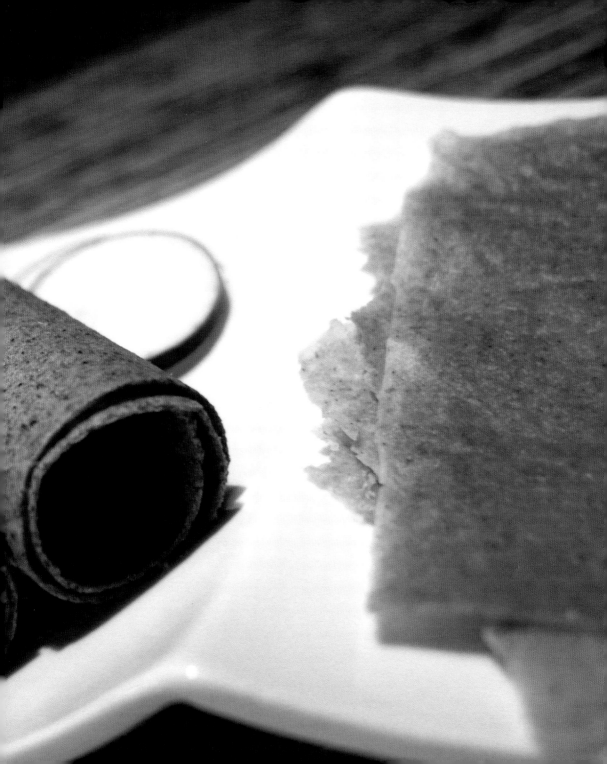

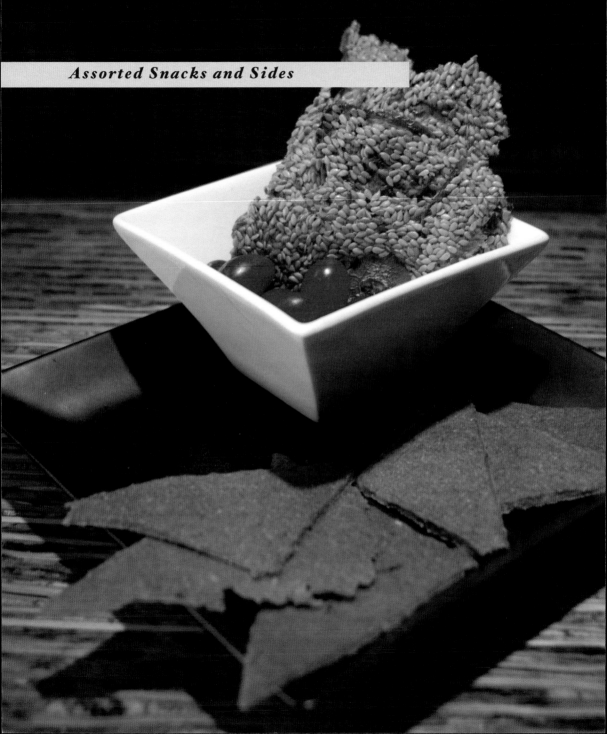

— SICILIAN FLAX CRACKERS —

These versatile flax crackers are enjoyable any time of the day as a snack and make great crusts. Inspired by rich Italian flavors, they're especially good with a layer of pesto and bruschetta!

4 cups soaked dark flaxseed (soaked at least 1 hour, but not more than 4 hours)
2 cups thinly sliced Roma tomatoes
1 cup Sun-Dried-Tomato Marinara (page 89)

In a large mixing bowl, combine marinara, sliced tomatoes, and gelatinous flax mixture. Toss well so that all ingredients combine. Spread out about ¼-inch thick over 2 covered dehydrator trays. Dehydrate at 110° for 12 hours until nice and crispy. To speed up dehydrating time, flip over after 8 hours. Gently break into pieces for use, or score about 2 hours into drying time to desired shape and size.

— CORN CHIPS —

These crispy chips will save in an airtight container indefinitely, but are best enjoyed in the first 30 days.

2 cups ground golden flaxseed
2 cups bicolor corn
2 cups water
2 Tbsp. chili powder
2 cloves garlic

Blend all ingredients in a high-powered blender until thick and well combined. Spread out evenly in ¼-inch layer over dehydrator tray. Using spatula, score into corn-chip shapes by dividing the tray in half, then in half again, in both directions. Afterward, split each square diagonally to achieve chip-like form. Dehydrate at 115° for 12 hours until crispy. To dehydrate faster, flip over after 8 hours.
Makes 32 chips.

— Rojo Salsa —

This deep-red salsa can be adapted to your own desired level of spice by the addition of more peppers to the mixture. The basic recipe is easy and can be prepared in less than 5 minutes. If you don't have a food processor, it can be prepared by hand, so this salsa makes for an easy recipe when on the road or short on time.

4 diced Roma tomatoes
2 cloves garlic
⅓ cup de-stemmed cilantro leaves
¼ cup chopped green onions
   (green and white portions of stalk)

1 tsp. Celtic sea salt
½ small serrano chili pepper, diced
Juice from 1 lime
Juice from 1 lemon

In food processor, combine garlic, cilantro, green onions, sea salt, chili pepper, and juice. Pulse until well mixed but still chunky. Add diced Roma tomato and pulse again until desired thickness is achieved. A light pulse will create a "pico de gallo"–style salsa, and a longer run will create more of a liquid. If you don't have a food processor, lightly chop all ingredients on a cutting board and slide into a medium mixing bowl. Toss well. Salsa lasts 3–4 days in the refrigerator.

Makes 2 cups.

— Spicy Tortillas —

These tortillas can be made in advance and keep for up to 15 days in the refrigerator. They're great for use in a variety of Mexican dishes, and they make a wonderful wrap overall.

2 cups sprouted Kamut grain (sprouted 3–5 days)
2 cups water
1 cup ground golden flaxseed
2 Tbsp. chili powder

2 Tbsp. cold-pressed extra-virgin olive oil
1 tsp. sea salt
1 Tbsp. psyllium husk
1 clove garlic

Rinse and drain sprouted grain. Blend all ingredients (except for psyllium husk) in a high-powered blender until a thick mixture forms. Add psyllium until mixture begins to congeal. Spread on covered dehydrator trays into 8-inch-round tortilla shapes. Dehydrate at 110° for 4 hours. Flip over and dehydrate an additional 20 minutes.

Makes 6 tortillas.

— GREEN GUACAMOLE —

Early on in my exploration of living foods, I (Jenny) found that certain ingredients complemented one another and also allowed for a higher level of nutrition in ordinary, everyday recipes. This guacamole is unusually rich in vitamin B_6 due to the dulse flakes and is delightfully salty as a result, but still low in sodium.

2 ripe Hass avocados
Juice of 1 lemon
$1/8$ cup de-stemmed cilantro leaves
1 chopped green onion (green and white portions of stalk)
1 Tbsp. dulse flakes
$1/2$ tsp. Himalayan salt
$1/2$ tsp. cayenne pepper (optional)

In medium-sized mixing bowl, combine lemon juice, cilantro leaves, green onion, dulse flakes, cayenne pepper, and Himalayan salt. Whisk together gently so all ingredients are lightly covered with juice. Add Hass avocados, and using a fork or a pestle, gently mash them into the lemon mixture until a slightly creamy texture forms. Use within 48 hours for best results.

Makes 2 cups.

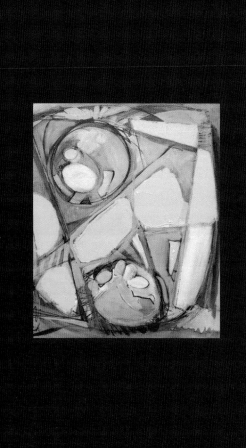

Chapter Six

Delicious,
Raw Living
Entrées

The entrée dishes at 118° use several different sauces, spreads, vegetables, and wraps. We suggest that you make the sauces first and then the individual entrées. Many of the sauces and wraps are interchangeable to give you a great amount of flexibility and room for creative expression in your own kitchen.

We encourage you to play with these recipes and make them your own. Enjoy the unique flavors that arise from using the wraps, sauces, and vegetables in combination—for example, in the Ensenada Enchiladas, Asian Infusion, and Topaz Pizza.

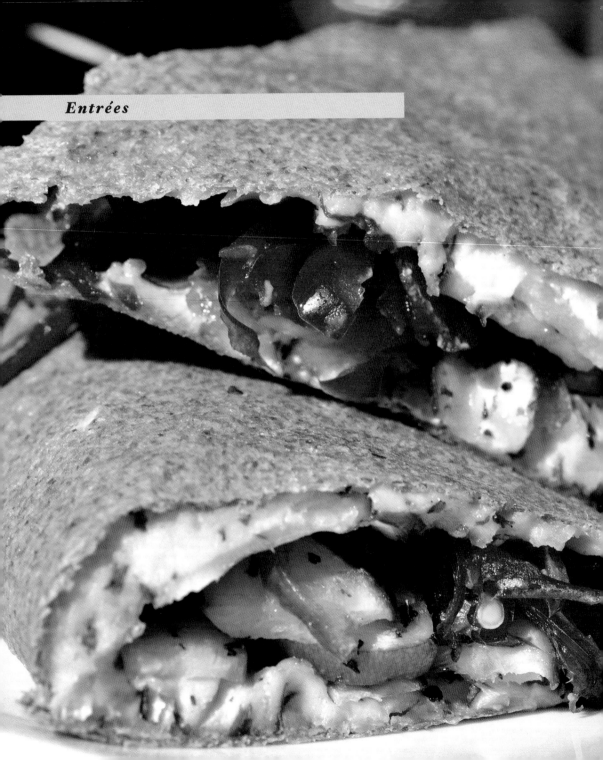

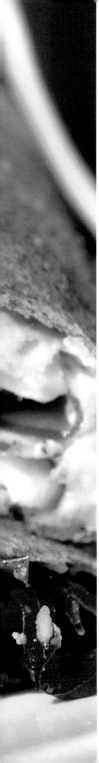

— HEIRLOOM-SQUASH SAMOSA —

Heirloom-variety vegetables are grown from ancient seeds that are thought to be the most natural, original versions of the plant and haven't been hybridized over the years. These varieties have proven to provide superior taste and nutritional value. This recipe is a protein-packed option that's easy for the body to break down and use quickly. It can be enjoyed any time of the day and is especially good warm from the dehydrator!

WRAP:
Use 1 tray Zucchini-Flax Wrap (page 96)

FILLING:
2 cups Tahini Cheese (page 81)
4 cups Italian-marinated heirloom squash
4 cups marinated red bell peppers
½ cup Red Bell Pepper Puree (page 87)

Begin by cutting Zucchini-Flax Wrap into 4 equal squares. Lightly spread a layer of Tahini Cheese over the top of each. Fill with marinated vegetables, and top with Red Bell Pepper Puree. Fold squares over into triangles. Cut each triangle into 2 equal pieces, and warm in dehydrator at 105° for 30–40 minutes. Enjoy!
Makes 4 servings.

— GARDEN TAHINI ROLLS —

This sushi-style roll offers a high concentration of omegas, protein, and fresh vegetables. This vibrant dish is a definite party pleaser. The Tahini Cheese also provides an extra boost of calcium, making this a nutritious meal any time of day.

WRAP:
Use 1 tray Zucchini-Flax Wrap (page 96)

FILLING:
½ cup Tahini Cheese (page 81)
2 medium-sized zucchini, julienned
1 large carrot, grated
2 red bell peppers, sliced thin
4 leaves kale, cut into thin strips

GARNISH:
¼ cup Red Bell Pepper Puree (page 87)

Prepare wrap by cutting 1 tray of Zucchini-Flax Wrap into 2 equal rectangular pieces. Gently spread ¼ cup Tahini Cheese on each wrap, beginning from the edge and working ¾ of the way up (leaving about ½ inch uncovered at the top for rolling), forming a thin layer of cheese. Additional cheese may be added as desired.

About ½ inch from the bottom of each wrap, line up carrots, dividing them evenly between wraps. Repeat with julienned squash and red bell peppers, and finish with kale.

Next, gently roll each wrap into a tight, long roll. Gently cut rolls in half and then repeat, so that you have 8 equal pieces per roll. Garnish with Red Bell Pepper Puree for additional flavor.

Makes 4 servings of 4 pieces.

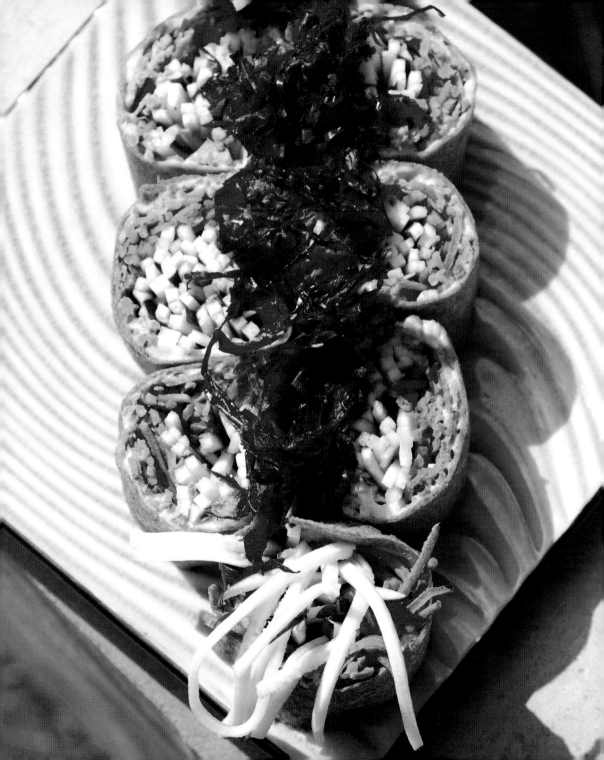

— TOPAZ PIZZA —

This recipe is a pizza lover's dream! Not only is the soft crust high in protein, but the delicious flavors of pesto and marinated vegetables make this dish a delight for the palate. Enjoyed warm right out of the dehydrator, this pizza practically melts in your mouth.

CRUST:
Use 4 triangles of Olive Kamut Bread (page 92)
(cut 1 tray of bread in half and cut each half into 2 squares;
further cut squares diagonally to get triangles)

TOPPING:
1 cup Pistachio Pesto (page 86)
4 Roma tomatoes, sliced thin
2 cups Italian-marinated squash
½ cup Basil Cheese (page 36)

GARNISH:
½ cup Sun-Dried-Tomato Marinara (page 89)

Spread a layer of Pistachio Pesto ¼-inch thick over each triangle of pizza crust. Layer with freshly cut tomato and ½ cup squash per slice, and sprinkle with crumbled Basil Cheese. Garnish with Sun-Dried-Tomato Marinara and enjoy!

Makes 4 servings.

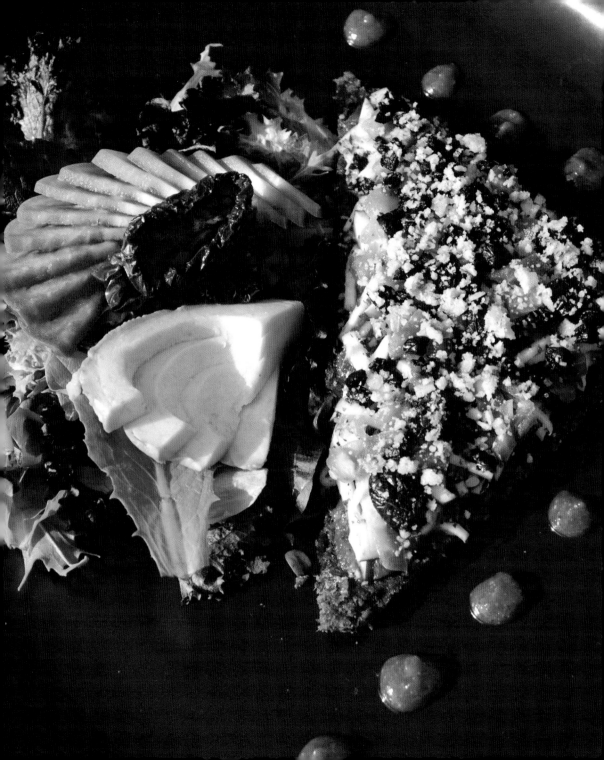

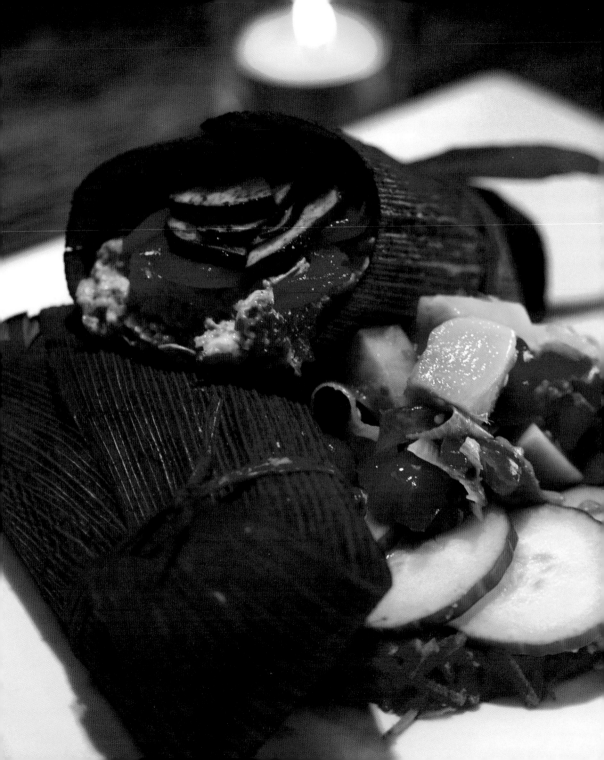

— SWEET CORN TAMALES —

Tamales were a popular dish when I (Jenny) was growing up in California. The mystique and excitement of unwrapping each one always evoked a sense of adventure at the beginning of the meal. These tamales are sweet and savory . . . and one of the most popular dishes at 118.

For this recipe, you'll need 12 large-sized corn husks, soaked in water until pliable.

TAMALE FILLING:
4 cups bicolor corn
2 cups pine nuts
1 Roma tomato
2 cloves garlic
2 Tbsp. chili powder
2 Tbsp. cold-pressed extra-virgin olive oil

TOPPING:
2 cups portobello mushrooms
1 cup Rojo Salsa (page 100)

Combine corn and pine nuts in a food processor and process until lightly broken down. Add tomato, garlic, chili powder, and olive oil and process into a thick paste.

Assemble soaked corn husks on cutting boards. Scoop a 2-inch ball of filling into the center of each husk, and then top with portobello mushrooms and salsa. Fold over and tie tamales. Place in dehydrator at 110° for 1–2 hours before enjoying. The longer they're in the dehydrator, the drier the filling will get.

Makes 4 servings.

— LIVING LASAGNA—

This is a rich and creamy lasagna that one 118 customer said could rival his Italian mother's version! We think it's pretty good, too!

The preparation of this recipe is done in layers, and for each one, you'll repeat a series of ingredients. This entrée can be layered on a dehydrator sheet if you're preparing it in the dehydrator, or in a glass pan if you're letting it marinate in the refrigerator.

LASAGNA:
4 large zucchini
4 large Roma tomatoes, thinly sliced
4 cups Macadamia-Spinach Ricotta (page 84)
1 cup Sun-Dried-Tomato Marinara (page 89)

GARNISH:
2 cups Sun-Dried Tomatoes (page 89)

Begin by slicing zucchini lengthwise on a mandoline set at $1/8$ inch. Each zucchini should yield 12–16 slices.

Layer 3 to 4 slices of zucchini, followed by 1 slice Roma tomato, and then a $1/2$-inch layer of ricotta and a drizzle of marinara per serving. Repeat, and finish the second layer with a slice of zucchini topped with a drizzle of marinara.

Dehydrate at 110° for 3–4 hours or until the cheese sets. Remove from dehydrator and sprinkle with Sun-Dried Tomatoes.

Makes 4 servings.

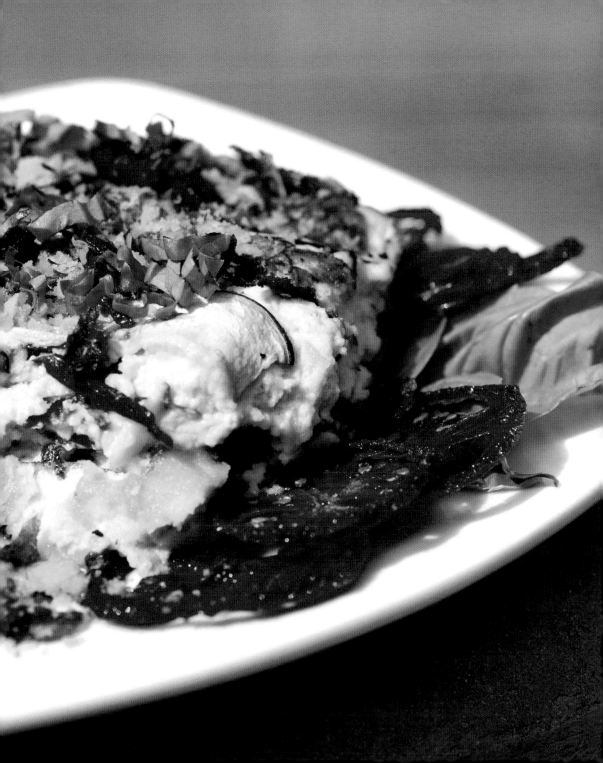

— Asian Infusion —

The discovery of this amazing pasta came in a divinely inspired moment while in search of the perfect balance of flavor and nutrition. This recipe is high in protein, iron, B vitamins, and trace minerals. In addition to being nutritious, the dish has a mellow, savory flavor that will be a tap dance for your taste buds! Enjoy!

4 zucchini, julienned
10 enoki mushrooms (¹⁄₈ cup fresh green onions can be substituted)
2 cups marinated portobello mushrooms
1 ripe Hass avocado
1 cup dulse
1½ cups Chipotle Cheese (page 83)
½ cups Miso Dressing (page 87)

Toss all ingredients well in a large mixing bowl until rich and creamy. Stack into a compression mold and fill until well packed. Invert, forming tower of mixture, and top with a sprinkling of enoki mushrooms for garnish.

Makes 4 servings.

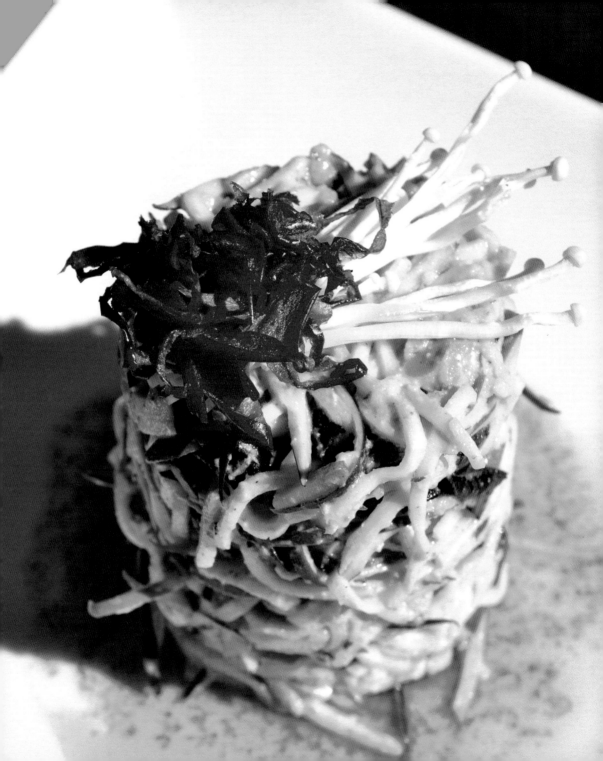

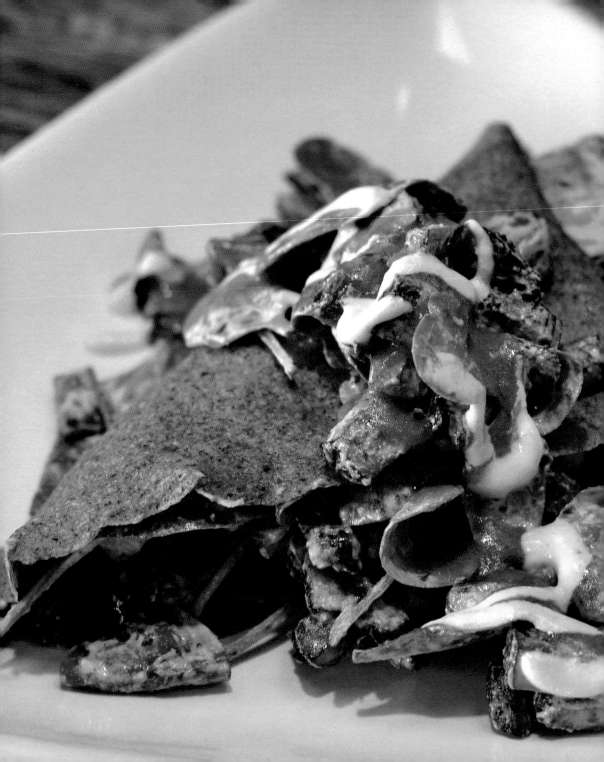

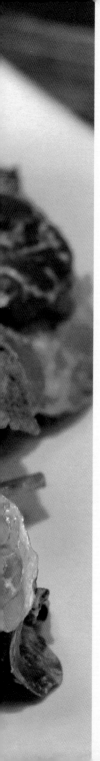

— MUSHROOM CREPES —

This recipe combines fresh spinach, mushrooms, and a rich garlic crème for a decadent dish that can be enjoyed in any season. These crepes were designed to incorporate fresh vegetables and offer a nice combination of textures. High in protein, the sprouted-grain wraps are deliciously delicate.

CREPE WRAP:

2 cups sprouted Kamut grain
(sprouted 3–5 days)
1½ cups water
¼ cup cold-pressed extra-virgin olive oil

1 Tbsp. dried Italian seasoning
1 tsp. agave nectar
1 tsp. Himalayan salt
2 Tbsp. psyllium husk

FILLING:

2 cups Garlic Crème Sauce (page 90)
4 cups marinated portobello mushrooms

4 cups chopped spinach
1 cup chopped fresh basil

Crepe-wrap preparation:

Rinse and drain sprouted grain. Blend all ingredients (except for psyllium husk) in a high-powered blender until well mixed, creamy, and thick. Add psyllium husk and blend for 20 seconds. Spread out evenly in a ⅛-inch-thick layer over 4 dehydrator trays covered in nonstick drying sheets, and dehydrate at 110° for 4 hours.

Filling preparation:

In a medium-sized mixing bowl, toss spinach and mushrooms with Garlic Crème Sauce. Add chopped basil to taste.

Assembly:

Cut crepe wrap into 4 equal squares and top each with ¼ of filling mixture. Fold over into rectangle, and cut on the diagonal into 2 long triangular pieces.

Makes 4 servings.

— RAW RAMEN BOWL —

This is a warm, filling entrée soup that's rich and creamy—and filled with fresh vegetables and superfoods!

BROTH:
- 4 cups warm or hot water
- 1 large zucchini
- 2 cups pine nuts
- Juice of 1 lemon
- 2 cloves garlic
- 1 tsp. Himalayan salt
- 1 Tbsp. miso paste
- 1 green onion
- 1 dash cayenne pepper
- 1 tsp. curry (optional)

SOUP TOPPING:
- ½ cup dulse pieces
- ½ cup chopped laver
- 2 cups julienned squash
- Coconut noodles (as desired)
- ¼ cup chopped green onions
- 1 avocado, cubed

Blend all broth ingredients well in a high-powered blender. Pour into two entrée-sized soup bowls. Top with desired topping ingredients and enjoy!

Makes 2 servings.

— MACADAMIA-COCONUT CURRY WRAP —

A luscious combination of fresh farmers'-market vegetables, creamy macadamia sauce, and a sweet curry wrap, this entrée is not only appealing to the eyes, but it invokes a healthy glow in your hair, skin, and nails!

WRAP:
Use 1 tray curry Coconut Wrap (page 94)

FILLING:
2 cups macadamia nuts
1 cup young Thai coconut water
1 cup young Thai coconut flesh
2 cloves garlic
1 red bell pepper
1 Roma tomato
Juice of 1 lemon
1 tsp. sea salt

FARMERS'-MARKET VEGETABLES:
2 cups thinly sliced red bell peppers
1 cup Spicy Spanish Squash (page 47)
2 leaves finely chopped red Swiss chard

GARNISH:
¼ cup Red Bell Pepper Puree
¼ cup chopped fresh basil

Blend all filling ingredients well in a high-powered blender until rich and creamy.

In a medium-sized mixing bowl, combine vegetables and filling, and toss well. Cut Coconut Wrap into four equal squares. Fill each square with ¼ of the mixture, and roll lengthwise. Garnish with Red Bell Pepper Puree and chopped basil.

Makes 4 servings.

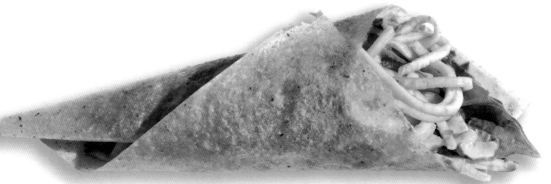

— BAJA BURRITO —

Baja Mexico is well known for its fresh fruit and subtropical climate. This burrito was inspired by the region's lush coastline and the hearty appetite that develops after a long day playing in the sunshine there.

WRAP:

Use 4 Spicy Tortillas (page 100)

FILLING:

2 cups Chipotle Cheese (page 83)
2 cups shredded carrots
2 cups mango, diced
2 cups chopped spinach
2 cups sliced cremini mushrooms
2 ripe Hass avocado, diced
½ cup fresh cilantro
¼ cup chopped green onions
1 Tbsp. chili powder
3 Tbsp. cold-pressed extra-virgin olive oil

GARNISH:

¼ cup Pine-Nut Sour Cream (page 86)
¼ cup Avocado-Lime Sauce (page 91)
¼ cup Red Bell Pepper Puree (page 87)

Toss all filling ingredients well in a medium-sized mixing bowl. Fill each tortilla with ¼ of mixture and roll tightly. Garnish each with Pine-Nut Sour Cream, Avocado-Lime Sauce, and Red Bell Pepper Puree. Add any remaining fresh cilantro or chopped green onions to the top.

Makes 4 servings.

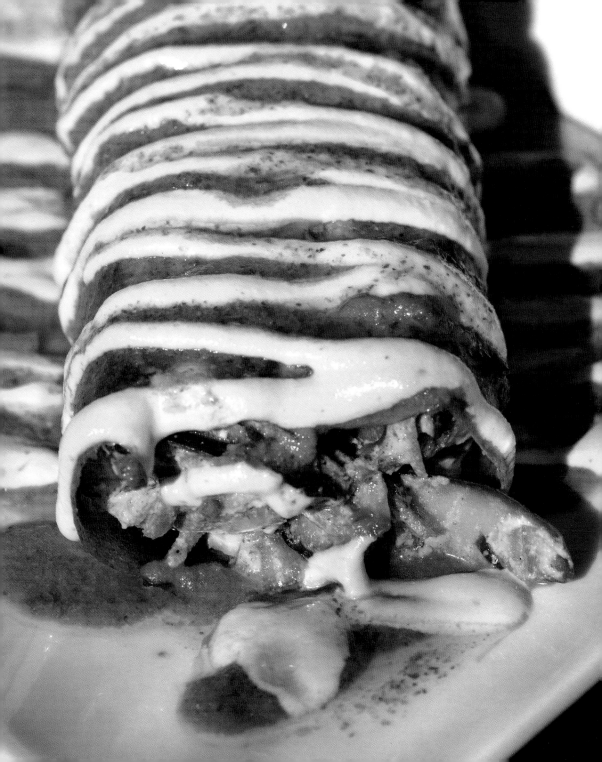

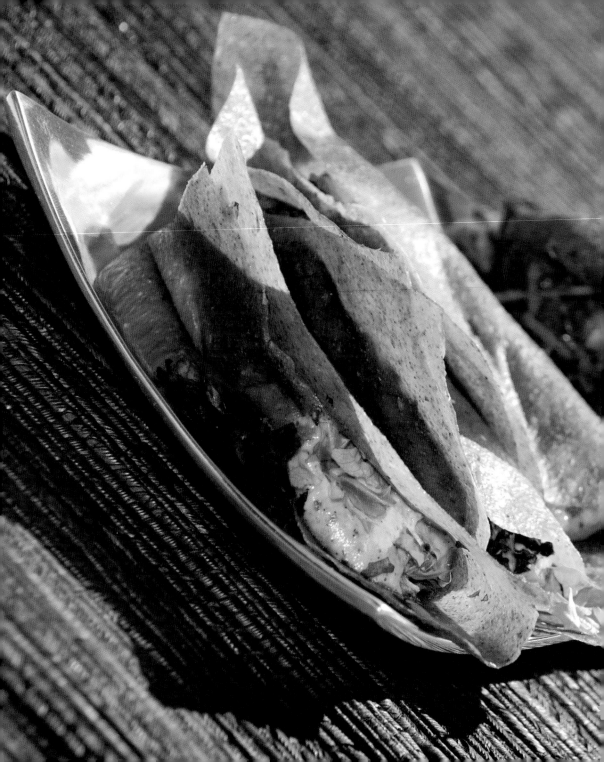

— CLAYUDAS —

In Oaxaca, Mexico, there's a traditional dish called *clayudas*: a large round corn tortilla topped with the freshest of daily vegetables, nopales (cactus), and cheeses. This version is a vibrant recipe that's great for optimal daily health. Cactus is widely known as a plant that can aid in the healing of all types of digestive distress.

SHELL:

2 cups sprouted buckwheat (sprouted 12 hours)
1 cup ground golden flaxseed
2 cups water
1 large Roma tomato
1 red bell pepper
1 tsp. sea salt
2 Tbsp. chili powder
1 clove garlic

TOPPING:

2 cups Avocado-Lime Sauce (page 91)
2 cups Chipotle Cheese (page 83)
2 cups bicolor corn
2 julienned cucumbers
1 cup chopped nopales (cactus)*
2 cups chopped spinach
2 cups avocado
2 cups Spicy Spanish Squash (page 47)

Shell preparation:

Rinse and drain sprouted buckwheat. Blend ingredients well, and spread in 7-inch rounds about ⅛-inch thick on covered dehydrator trays. Dehydrate at 110° for 8 hours until crispy. Makes 6 shells.

Assembly:

In a medium-sized mixing bowl, toss the Chipotle Cheese, corn, cactus, spinach, and avocado. Spread a thin layer of Avocado-Lime Sauce and 1 cup of vegetable mixture over clayudas shell, and top with julienned cucumber. Makes 6 servings.

*For nopales, de-thorn and dice into ¼-inch pieces. Marinate in lemon juice and sea salt (will save for 7 days after prepared in this manner).

— NEW AGE QUESADILLA —

When I (Jenny) was younger, coming home to a fresh quesadilla was my favorite treat. This one is the perfect combination of sweet and spicy, and can be enjoyed by people of all ages—a few minutes in the dehydrator to warm is all it takes. Simply prepare a batch of the tortillas in advance and fill with the fresh vegetable mixture.

TORTILLAS:
  Use 4 Spicy Tortillas (page 100)

VEGETABLE MIXTURE:
  2 cups Almond Cheese (page 82)
  4 cups chopped spinach
  2 cups bicolor corn
  2 ripe avocados
  2 cups chopped peppers

GARNISH:
  1 cup Rojo Salsa (page 100)
  2 cups Green Guacamole (page 101)

Begin by laying out 4 tortillas on a flat cutting-board surface. In a medium-sized mixing bowl, toss vegetables with Almond Cheese until well mixed. Fill each tortilla with ¼ of filling and gently fold over. Place in dehydrator at 115° for 10–15 minutes to warm. Top each quesadilla with ¼ cup Rojo Salsa and ½ cup Green Guacamole and enjoy!

  Makes 4 servings.

— Ensenada Enchiladas —

We both frequently traveled Baja Mexico to scuba dive its serene waters. Along the way, we always enjoyed the mellow flavors of the local produce.

When I (Jenny) first learned about living foods, I became even more inspired by the vibrant colors of the produce along the coastline and the subtle Spanish flavors unique to this area of Mexico. This recipe was inspired by a particularly bright and beautiful day on my last trip down, with just the perfect amount of ocean breeze to tickle your toes.

WRAP:
Use 1 tray tomato Coconut Wrap (page 94)

FILLING:
6 cups Spicy Spanish Squash (page 47)
3 cups marinated portobello mushrooms
1¼ cups bicolor corn
1 large carrot, shredded
3 ripe avocados, sliced
1¼ cup Chipotle Cheese (page 83)

TOPPING:
1 cup Avocado-Lime Sauce (page 91)
1 cup Red Bell Pepper Puree (page 87)
1 cup Sweet Cheese (page 82)
1 cup Rojo Salsa (page 100)

Begin by cutting tomato Coconut Wrap into 6 equal pieces by first cutting in half, and then cutting each half into 3 equal pieces. Lay out on a flat work surface. Layer vegetables in the middle of each wrap: squash first, then mushrooms, corn, carrots, and avocado. Top with 2–4 Tbsp. Chipotle Cheese per enchilada.

Gently roll up each enchilada and top with Avocado-Lime Sauce, Red Bell Pepper Puree, Sweet Cheese, and Rojo Salsa.

Makes 6 scrumptious servings!

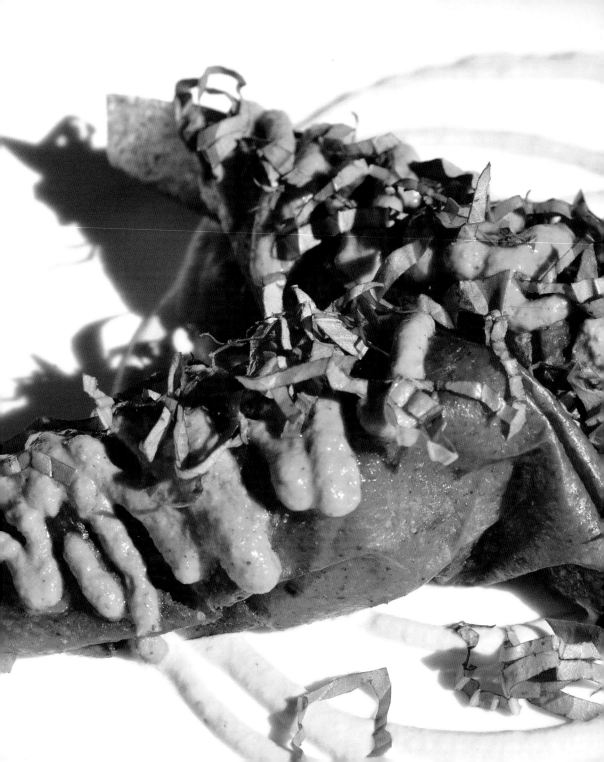

— PESTO TORTELLINI —

These tortellini are a dinner favorite at 118. The delicate wraps make this dish especially rich, and the filling is a savory treat. Delight your friends at your next dinner party with this recipe, which is guaranteed to knock their socks off. The flavors of basil, garlic, and olive oil are especially enjoyable.

WRAP:
Use 1 tray basil Coconut Wrap (page 94)

FILLING:
2 cups julienned yellow crookneck squash or zucchini
1 cup shredded carrots
1 cup thinly sliced red bell peppers
2 cups Pistachio Pesto (page 86)
1 cup Sun-Dried-Tomato Marinara (page 89)

GARNISH:
1 cup Basil Cheese (page 36)
½ cup Sun-Dried-Tomato Marinara (page 89)

Begin by cutting sheet of basil Coconut Wrap in half lengthwise. Cut each half into 4 equal portions. Line up all 8 pieces on cutting board. In a medium-sized mixing bowl, toss filling ingredients together until well combined. Fill each tortellini shell with ⅛ of mixture.

Gently fold each shell over to form a tortellini. Place all 8 pieces into dehydrator at 115° for 20 minutes. Transfer from dehydrator onto a plate, and top with marinara and Basil Cheese.

Makes 2 entrée-sized servings or 4 appetizer servings.

— BUTTERNUT-SQUASH RAVIOLI —

Butternut squash is a wonderful seasonal selection that makes these ravioli a decadent treat. Inspired by the change of season, with the wonderful warming flavors of rosemary, these ravioli are a favorite recipe to prepare and enjoy with family and friends.

RAVIOLI WRAP:
Use 2 trays basil Coconut Wrap (page 94)

FILLING:
4 cups cubed butternut squash
½ cup cold-pressed extra-virgin olive oil
¼ cup pine nuts
1 Roma tomato
2 cloves garlic
1 sprig rosemary

1 Tbsp. agave nectar
1 tsp. sea salt
1 tsp. dried Italian seasoning
1 cup water
2 cups chopped portobello mushrooms
2 cups Italian-marinated squash

GARNISH:
½ cup Red Bell Pepper Puree (page 87)
1 cup Crispy Tomatoes (page 41)

Preparation of filling:
Combine all ingredients (except for mushrooms and Italian squash) in high-powered blender. Blend well and pour mixture into medium-sized bowl. Add mushrooms and marinated squash and toss well.

Assembly:
Cut each tray of basil Coconut Wraps into 3 pieces, and then cut each of those into 3 squares, totaling 9 per tray. Fill squares with 2 Tbsp. of filling each and gently fold over into triangular pieces. Set in dehydrator at 110° (using the dehydrator screen) for 40–60 minutes, and allow the filling to set. Remove from dehydrator and serve over spinach. Garnish with Red Bell Pepper Puree and Crispy Tomatoes.

Makes 4 servings of 4 ravioli each.

— LEMON-PESTO PASTA —

This pasta is a great beginner recipe and is fun to prepare with kids of all ages. It's a lunch favorite at 118 and can be made three to four days in advance and enjoyed throughout the week (especially if you don't salt the dish during preparation but instead wait until it's served, since salt causes the water to separate from the starch in the squash, creating excess liquid in the dish).

4 zucchini and/or yellow crookneck squash, julienned on a mandoline or using a spiralizing machine
4 cups Pistachio Pesto (page 86)
2 cups Sun-Dried-Tomato Marinara (page 89)
2 cups portobello mushrooms, diced
2 cups chopped basil

Toss pasta with pesto, marinara, mushrooms, and basil. Top with your choice of Sun-Dried Tomato (page 89), Basil Cheese (page 36), or fresh olives.
Makes 4 servings.

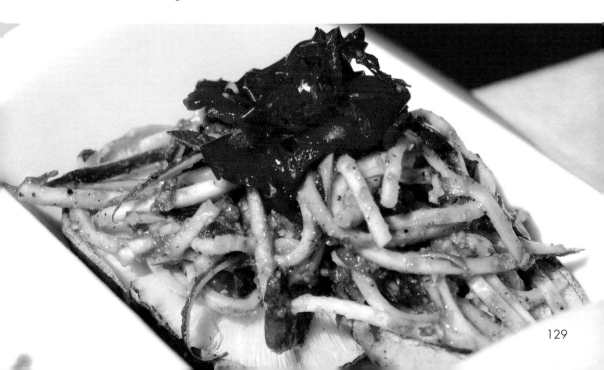

— SWEET CRÈME PIZZA —

This pizza was introduced on 118's special brunch menu and has become a mainstay ever since. The recipe is best enjoyed warm from the dehydrator and is a great all-around dish to serve to guests. The flavors of the sweet crème and marinated vegetables together make for a mouthwatering treat that's also high in protein and calcium.

CRUST:
Use 4 triangles of Olive Kamut Bread (page 92)
   (cut 1 tray of bread in half and cut each half into 2 squares;
    further cut squares diagonally to get triangles)

TOPPING:
2 cups Sweet Cheese (page 82)
1 cup marinated red bell peppers
1 cup marinated portobello mushrooms
1 cup marinated Italian squash

GARNISH:
¼ cup chopped sun-dried black olives
¼ cup chopped fresh basil

In a medium-sized mixing bowl, combine Sweet Cheese and marinated red bell peppers, portobello mushrooms, and Italian squash. Toss until well mixed. Split topping mixture into 4 equal portions, and top each triangle. Place triangles in dehydrator at 110° for 2 hours. The cheese will set and the pizza will warm. Sprinkle with olives and basil before serving and enjoy!

Makes 4 servings.

— Sweet-Onion Panini —

Paninis are traditionally thin grilled sandwiches, popular in Mediterranean communities. Ours is a wonderful living expression of savory marinated vegetables, sweet garlic cream cheese, and flavorful bread. This sandwich is packed with protein from the sprouted grains and fresh vegetables. Enjoy at a picnic in the park—these sandwiches travel well and are great for long trips!

Bread:
Use 1 sheet Onion Poppy-Seed Bread (page 93)

Vegetable filling:
2 cups marinated red bell peppers
2 cups marinated portobello mushrooms
2 cups marinated Italian squash
4 Roma tomatoes, thinly sliced
2 cups fresh, cleaned spinach
¼ cup Sweet Garlic Cream Cheese (see below for preparation)

Cut sheet of bread into 4 equal squares. Further cut each square diagonally into 2 separate pieces so that you have 8 triangles. Spread ⅛-inch layer of garlic cream cheese over triangles. Layer with tomato slices, spinach, and marinated vegetables.

Makes 4 sandwiches (cut each triangle in half to serve).

— Sweet Garlic Cream Cheese —

1 cup pine nuts
Juice from 2 lemons
2 Tbsp. cold-pressed extra-virgin olive oil

1 tsp. sea salt
3 cloves garlic

Blend ingredients in a high-powered blender until rich and creamy.

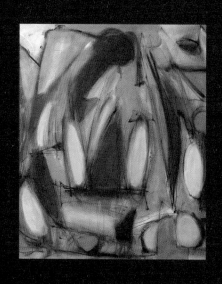

Chapter Seven

Sweet, Savory, and Healthful Desserts

Now you can eat dessert while maintaining a health-conscious lifestyle! These delicious treats are sure to satisfy even the most discriminating palate. Your children will enjoy the pleasures and health benefits of eating naturally sweetened desserts as well.

These desserts have served as staples at 118 and are popular with both adults and kids of all backgrounds.

Basic Sauces

The best desserts include a terrific sauce. These basic recipes provide the bases for many of the treats in this chapter and serve as an excellent garnish. (For all recipes except the Strawberry Sauce, you may need to scrape the sides of the blender to make sure ingredients are well mixed.) Feel free to make them in large batches to save for up to 10 days' worth of decadent desserts!

— Cinnamon Sauce —

1 cup agave nectar
1 Tbsp. cinnamon

1 drop cinnamon essential oil
1 dash sea salt

Place all ingredients in a high-powered blender and blend until rich and creamy in consistency. Once blended, transfer to a squeeze-bottle container with a standard tip to make garnishing fast and easy, or place in a sealed glass jar and store refrigerated for up to 10 days. Makes 1 cup.

— Chocolate Sauce —

3 cups raw cacao nibs or 2 cups raw cacao powder
1 tsp. vanilla extract or raw vanilla powder or 5 vanilla beans
¼ cup coconut oil

1 tsp. cinnamon
2 cups agave nectar
1 tsp. Himalayan salt

Place all ingredients in a high-powered blender and blend until rich and creamy in consistency. Once blended, transfer to a squeeze-bottle container with a standard tip to make garnishing fast and easy, or place in a sealed glass jar and store refrigerated for up to 10 days. Add 1 cup nut milk (see page 17 for recipes) to create a creamy texture and taste. Makes 2½ cups.

— Mint Sauce —

2 cups pine nuts
1 cup young Thai coconut water
½ cup agave nectar

¼ cup fresh mint leaves or 1 Tbsp. mint extract
1 tsp. sea salt

Place all ingredients in a high-powered blender and blend until rich and creamy in consistency. Once blended, transfer to a squeeze-bottle container with a standard tip to make garnishing fast and easy, or place in a sealed glass jar and store refrigerated for up to 10 days. Makes 2 cups.

— STRAWBERRY SAUCE —

8 oz. strawberries   2 Tbsp. agave nectar

Prepare strawberries by slicing off tops and rinsing well. In a high-powdered blender, blend with agave nectar into a nice puree. Makes 2 cups.

— CARAMEL SAUCE —

2 cups agave nectar   1 tsp. nutmeg   2 tsp. cinnamon
1 Tbsp. lucuma powder   1 tsp. ginger spice   1 dash sea salt
1 Tbsp. mesquite powder   1 tsp. clove spice
1 Tbsp. maca-root powder

Place all ingredients in a high-powered blender and blend until rich and creamy in consistency. Once blended, transfer to a squeeze-bottle container with a standard tip to make garnishing fast and easy, or place in a sealed glass jar and store refrigerated for up to 10 days. (You can use 1 Tbsp. pumpkin-pie spice as a substitute for the cinnamon, nutmeg, and other spices.) Makes 2 cups.

— VANILLA SAUCE —

2 Tbsp. vanilla extract or 4 vanilla beans   2 cups pine nuts   ¾ cup agave nectar
1 cup young Thai coconut water   1 dash Himalayan salt

Place all ingredients in a high-powered blender and blend until rich and creamy in consistency. Once blended, transfer to a squeeze-bottle container with a standard tip to make garnishing fast and easy, or place in a sealed glass jar and store refrigerated for up to 10 days. Makes 2 cups.

Dessert Bases

These delicious bases are used in many of the ice-cream, bar, cake, cookie, and truffle recipes in this chapter.

— ICE CREAM BASE —

4 cups pine nuts
2 cups young Thai coconut water
2 cups young Thai coconut flesh
2 cups agave nectar

Blend all ingredients well in a high-speed blender until thick and creamy. Makes 4 cups.

— MACADAMIA BAR BASE —

4 cups macadamia nuts (soaked 8 hours)
2½ cups agave nectar
1 Tbsp. lucuma powder (maca-root powder can be substituted)
1 tsp. sea salt
1 Tbsp. vanilla extract or 4 vanilla beans

Rinse and drain soaked macadamia nuts. Place all ingredients in a food processor and puree. Pour or spread over a dehydrator tray about ½-inch thick. Dehydrate at 110° for 12 hours. Makes 1 tray of bars.

— CHOCOLATE BASE —

2 cups cacao powder
1 tsp. vanilla extract
1 cup coconut oil

1 tsp. cinnamon
1 cup agave nectar
1 tsp. sea salt

Blend all ingredients in high-powered blender using the plunger to make sure mixture is well combined. Then pour into a medium-sized glass bowl and refrigerate for up to 2 hours to set. Makes 2 cups.

— NUT-FLOUR BASE —

8 cups almonds, pistachios, Brazil nuts, or macadamia nuts,
    depending on recipe or preference (soaked 4 hours)
8 cups water

Rinse and drain soaked nuts. Blend 4 cups nuts with 4 cups water. Repeat. Milk mixture through a nut-milk bag. Take remaining nut meal and dehydrate at 115° for 12 hours. Grind into flour and place in an airtight container. (Reserve milk for other recipes. This is a great use of extra sprouted nuts, allowing you to save the flour for an extended period of time without the nuts going bad.) Makes about 4 cups.

Sweet and Savory Desserts

— CHOCOLATE GANACHE SUPERFOOD SNACK —

Chocolate ganache has become a favorite at 118. Its rich superfood properties make it a balanced dessert that offers you sustained energy for the whole day. It's a great way to get your greens and other healthful superfoods while still enjoying the decadence of chocolate. If you have chocolate sensitivities, we recommend substituting carob powder in this recipe.

4 cups Chocolate Sauce (page 134)	1 Tbsp. spirulina	½ cup hemp seeds
3 Tbsp. maca-root powder	1 tsp. cinnamon	

Blend sauce, maca, and spirulina well in a high-powered blender until rich and creamy. Pour into a 8-inch-square tray and top with cinnamon and hemp seeds. Freeze for one hour and cut into desired shape.

This snack is great for kids and can be cut just like cookies into stars, hearts, and other fun shapes! Enjoy a 2" × 2" square for a great breakfast kick start to your day. Makes 16 pieces.

— ALMOND-BUTTER CUPS —

This is a healthy version of the classic peanut-butter-and-chocolate candy!

4 cups Chocolate Sauce (page 134)	2 cups raw almond butter	1 Tbsp. cinnamon
2 cups Almond Milk (page 17)	1 cup agave nectar	

In a large bowl, combine almond butter, agave, and cinnamon with a whisk until well mixed. Set aside.

Blend Chocolate Sauce with Almond Milk until creamy. Line up 2-inch-round small confectioner's cups. Fill ⅓ with chocolate mixture, ⅓ with almond-butter mixture, and final ⅓ with more chocolate mixture. Freeze 1 hour, serve, and enjoy! Makes 12 cups.

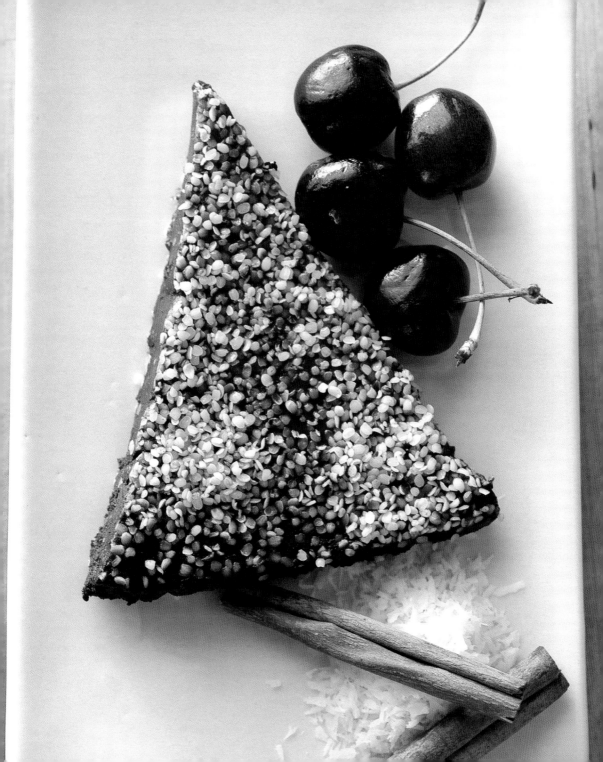

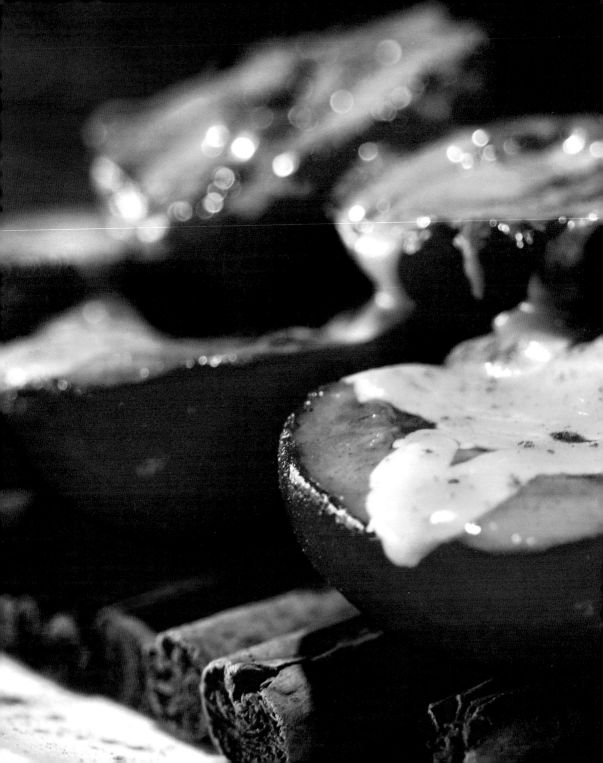

— PEACHES AND CREAM —

A creamy delight that works well for entertaining, this dessert is wonderful served warm and makes a delicious breakfast when topped with granola. These versatile natural cups of goodness are treats from Mother Nature!

2 cups Vanilla Sauce (page 135)
1 cup Cinnamon Sauce (page 134)
6 peaches, cut in half
1 cup agave nectar
1 tsp. cinnamon
1 pinch nutmeg

Blend agave, cinnamon, and nutmeg. Pour agave-spice mixture over peaches and place in dehydrator. Dehydrate at 110° for 4 hours.

Fill peach halves with 1 Tbsp. Vanilla Sauce, and drizzle with Cinnamon Sauce. Serve with a spoon.

Makes 6 servings.

— RASPBERRY CHEESECAKE —

This no-crust version of the classic cheesecake is rich, creamy, and oh-so-delicious!

2 cups macadamia nuts (soaked 8 hours)
1 Tbsp. vanilla extract or 3 vanilla beans
4 oz. raspberries, rinsed and drained

3 Tbsp. lemon juice
1 cup agave nectar
1 cup purified water

Rinse and drain soaked macadamia nuts. Blend all ingredients (except raspberries), pour into a 10-inch springform cake pan, and freeze one hour. In a small bowl, gently smash raspberries. Pour over cheesecake, and cut cake into slices. *Optional:* sprinkle unsweetened coconut shreds into the pan before freezing to create a crust-like bottom.
Makes 10 slices.

— NEAPOLITAN PARFAIT —

This recipe is easy to create once you've prepared the dessert sauces. Children love to make and eat this parfait, which is also a favorite treat to present at dinner parties. Your guests will be dazzled—and they won't know how easy it was to make!

8 oz. fresh strawberries, chopped
2 cups Vanilla Sauce (page 135)

2 cups Strawberry Sauce (page 135)
2 cups Chocolate Sauce (page 134)

In fluted glasses, layer as follows:
⅓ Vanilla Sauce
⅓ Chocolate Sauce
⅓ Strawberry Sauce

As you layer, smooth with a spoon to make even. Top with fresh strawberries.
Makes 4 servings.

— Cappuccino Crème Brûlée —

This is a great dessert for those who are new to raw foods, offering a familiar flavor and aroma. This recipe has a brilliant, velvety texture and makes a nice presentation if served in cappuccino cups straight from the freezer. This is a great finish to any Italian meal and may motivate you to sit and talk for hours with good friends.

2 cups pine nuts
1 cup young Thai coconut flesh
2 cup young Thai coconut water
1 cup agave nectar

2 shots espresso
½ tsp. Himalayan salt
½ tsp. cinnamon
1 Tbsp. psyllium husk

Blend all ingredients (except psyllium husk) in a high-powered blender. Add psyllium husk and blend for an additional 30 seconds. Pour mixture into small cappuccino cups. Let set in freezer for 1 hour. Remove and garnish with fresh raspberries.

Makes 4 servings.

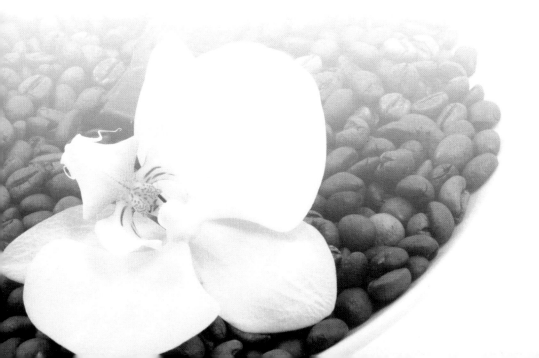

— CINNAMON FIGS AND CHEESE —

When figs are ripe and in season, this recipe shines! There's nothing like a beautiful, plump fig—the flavor bursts in your mouth—and in this dessert the creamy, rich texture is just perfect. This platter is a customer favorite at 118, and we know that it will quickly become a favorite in your home as well.

FIGS:
8 oz. figs, cut in half
4 Tbsp. Cinnamon Sauce (page 134)
2 Tbsp. Vanilla Sauce (page 135)

CHEESE:
2 cups raw ground-sesame tahini
1 cup lemon juice
1 Tbsp. Himalayan salt
¼ cup green onions, chopped

In a food processor, combine cheese ingredients into a thick, spreadable consistency.

Cut figs and remove stems. Roll in Cinnamon Sauce until well coated. Spread ¼-inch-thick dollop of cheese over figs and place facedown on nonstick drying sheet. Spread remaining cheese ¼-inch thick on drying sheet, to be used as garnish. Dehydrate at 105° for 1 hour.

Serve figs (with the cut side facing upward) with cheese lightly crumbled over the top. Garnish with Vanilla Sauce. Makes 6–8 servings.

— DATE-AND-CHEESE PLATTER —

Savory desserts make a nice break from anything too sweet and are great for those with sugar sensitivities. This platter is an easy dish to prepare and take to potlucks or picnics. Try using exotic organic dates like the rich, moist medjool variety.

DATES:
    6 dates

CHEESE:
2 cups pine nuts	1½ cups water
1 Tbsp. nutritional yeast	1 tsp. sea salt
2 cloves garlic	1 Roma tomato

Cheese preparation:

Blend cheese ingredients well in a high-powered blender, and spread over a nonstick drying sheet, forming a ¼-inch layer. Dehydrate at 115° for 6 hours.

Assembly:

Cut dates lengthwise after carefully removing their pits. Slice cheese into 4" x 3" rectangular pieces. Layer on a platter and serve. Makes 6 servings.

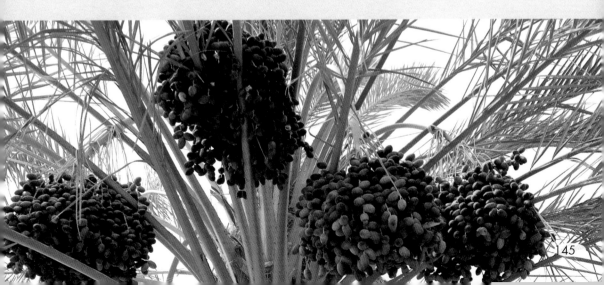

— SWEET BREAD AND PEPPERCORN CHEESE —

European travels inspired this recipe. In Europe, sweet breads abound. Usually paired with cheeses, they're absolutely perfect in the late afternoon while relaxing on an outdoor patio or socializing with friends and neighbors. Enjoy this recipe with fresh fruits of all kinds. The great thing is that what you don't finish will always save for tomorrow, so take some time to relax, sit back, and enjoy the sweet side of life.

PEPPERCORN CHEESE:

2 cups pine nuts (soaked 2 hours)
1 tsp. sea salt
1 Tbsp. nutritional yeast
2 Tbsp. lemon juice

1 Tbsp. agave nectar
3 Tbsp. psyllium husk
2 cups water

SWEET BREAD:

2 cups soaked, sprouted Kamut grain (sprouted 3–5 days)
½ cup agave nectar
2 tsp. Himalayan salt
Olive oil as needed (about ¼ cup)

Cheese preparation:

Rinse and drain soaked pine nuts. Blend all ingredients (except psyllium husk) in a blender until rich and creamy. Add psyllium until thick. Line a 4-inch circular mold with fresh peppercorn. Pour in cheese and refrigerate 4 hours. Remove, and invert mold.

Sweet-bread preparation:

Combine ingredients in a food processor. As the machine breaks down the Kamut, begin adding olive oil and agave nectar slowly until a clump of dough forms. Once it begins to stick to itself completely, the mixture is ready.

Line a cutting board with nonstick drying sheets. Wrap a rolling pin in plastic wrap (or use a nonstick rolling pin) and roll over dough to press it out flat into a sheet about ¼-inch thick. Place in dehydrator at 110° for 6 hours until soft and pliable but not crispy. Flip over and dehydrate an additional hour until dry to the touch. Cut into triangles and serve with cheese.

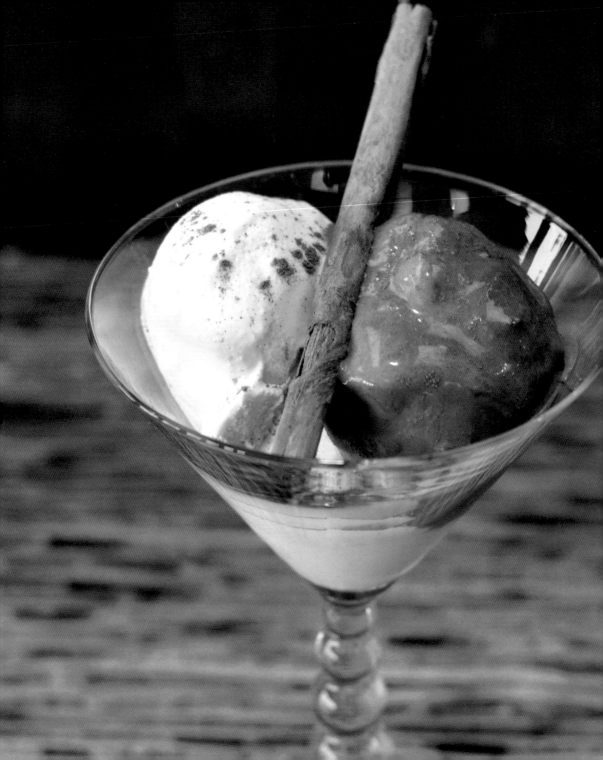

Ice Cream

These simple recipes for raw ice cream don't require an ice-cream maker. Simply blend, freeze, and enjoy!

— VANILLA GELATO —

4 cups Ice Cream Base (page 136)   1 tsp. Himalayan salt
3 Tbsp. vanilla

Blend all ingredients well in a blender until rich and creamy. Freeze immediately for 3 hours. Top with fresh berry puree and whole berries. Makes 4 cups.

— CHOCOLATE MINT —

4 cups Ice Cream Base (page 136)   3 Tbsp. coconut oil
1 cup raw cacao nibs   1 cup mint (fresh leaves)

Blend until thick and creamy. Sprinkle in cacao nibs. Stir, and freeze 3 hours. Makes 4 cups.

— CHAI CRÈME —

4 cups Ice Cream Base (page 136)   1 dash clove spice
1 Tbsp. cinnamon   3 Tbsp. mesquite powder
1 tsp. nutmeg   1 tsp. sea salt
1 tsp. ginger spice

Blend all ingredients well. Freeze 3 hours. You can substitute 1 Tbsp. pumpkin-pie spice for the other spices. Makes 4 cups.

Dessert Bars

Dessert bars are great options for parties and events. They're prepared one tray at a time and cut into the desired size. Easy to make . . . and, of course, to enjoy!

— TOFFEE BARS —

1 sheet Macadamia Bar Base (page 136) 8 oz. Cinnamon Sauce (page 134)
1 cup Chocolate Sauce (page 134) 8 oz. Caramel Sauce (page 135)

Spread chocolate evenly across the top of the bars with offset spatula. Place cinnamon and caramel in squeeze bottles. Create a pattern of crisscrossing lines across chocolate. Chill and cut into bars to serve. Makes 16 bars.

— LEMON-POMEGRANATE BARS —

1 sheet Macadamia Bar Base (page 136) 2 cups lemon juice 2 cups agave nectar
2 cups young Thai coconut flesh 4 Tbsp. psyllium husk

Blend lemon juice, coconut flesh, and agave nectar in a high-powered blender until creamy and smooth. Add psyllium husk until mixture begins to thicken (usually about 30 seconds). Spread evenly over bars. Sprinkle with fresh pomegranate seeds. (You can also substitute fresh berries for the seeds.) Makes 16 bars.

— CINNAMON-FIG BARS —

1 sheet Macadamia Bar Base (page 136) 1 Tbsp. cinnamon 1 tsp. nutmeg
4 cups fresh figs 1 tsp. sea salt 1 cup agave nectar

Blend agave, cinnamon, sea salt, and nutmeg. Dice figs and cover with agave-spice sauce mixture. Place in dehydrator at 115° for 4 hours. Remove mixture and stir. Spread evenly over bars. Makes 16 bars.

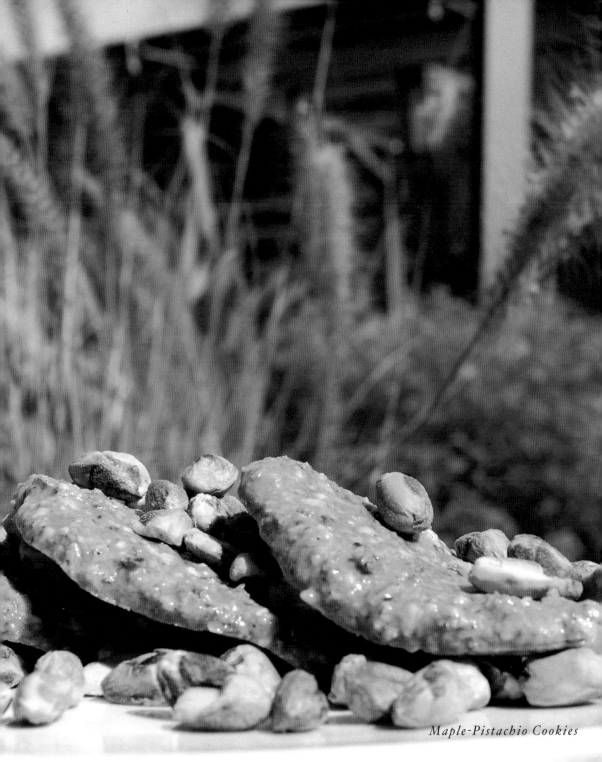

Maple-Pistachio Cookies

Cookies

Cookies are great to grab on the run and also make excellent breakfast options. Serve them with raw living ice cream, or take them on your next hike. They last indefinitely, but who can leave an excellent raw cookie lying around?

— MAPLE-PISTACHIO COOKIES —

4 cups pistachios
2 cups agave nectar
1 Tbsp. mesquite powder
1 Tbsp. cinnamon

1 tsp. nutmeg
1 tsp. ginger spice
1 tsp. Himalayan salt

Process pistachios in a food processor until coarsely fine. Blend the remaining ingredients in a blender. Add the liquid to the pistachios and process until a ball of dough forms. Roll out into large sheet and refrigerate for 1 hour.

Remove from refrigerator and cut into desired shapes. Makes 12–16 cookies.

— APPLE-CINNAMON-FIG-PECAN COOKIES —

2 ripe red or Fuji apples
2 cups pecans (soaked 6 hours)
2 cups dried figs (soaked 1 hour)

1 Tbsp. cinnamon
1 tsp. sea salt

Slice apples into ¼-inch-thick rounds and set aside. In a food processor, combine pecans, figs, cinnamon, and salt. Process until dough ball forms. On a covered dehydrator tray, begin by placing apple rounds ½ inch apart across tray. Scoop out dough mixture into 2-inch balls and place on top of apples. Gently press down into flat cookie shape. (*Tip:* Dip your fingers in water before pressing down so that mixture doesn't stick to them.) Dehydrate at 115° for 10 hours. Makes 12–16 cookies.

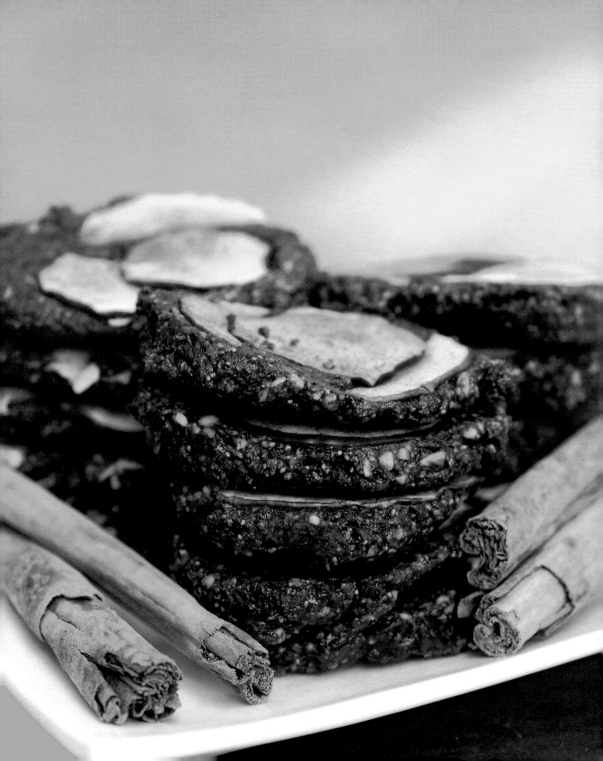

— CHOCOLATE-CHIP COOKIES —

COOKIE DOUGH:
4 cups Nut-Flour Base (use almonds—see page 137)
1½ cups agave nectar
2 tsp. cinnamon
1 tsp. sea salt
1 tsp. vanilla extract

CHOCOLATE CHIPS:
2 cups cacao nibs
½ cup agave nectar
1 Tbsp. vanilla extract or 4 vanilla beans

Preparation of dough:
Blend ingredients until creamy. Place in refrigerator about ½ hour to set.

Preparation of chocolate chips:
Blend agave and vanilla. Pour over nibs until well coated. Place in dehydrator at 110° for 2 hours.

Assembly:
Take chilled dough and form into 2-inch balls. Press down to flatten into circles. Press chocolate chips into each cookie. Dehydrate at 110° for 4 hours.
Makes 12–16 cookies.

— PIGNOLIA ITALIAN COOKIES —

COOKIE DOUGH:
4 cups Nut-Flour Base (use Brazil nuts—see page 137)
2 cups agave nectar
1 cup water
½ cup cold-pressed extra-virgin olive oil
1 tsp. Himalayan salt
2 tsp. cinnamon

TOPPING:
2 cups pine nuts (soaked 2–4 hours)
2 Tbsp. cinnamon
½ cup agave nectar

Preparation of dough:

In a bowl, combine nut flour, cinnamon, and salt. In a blender, combine agave, water, and oil. Put into bowl with flour mixture and smash together with your hands into dough. Roll out onto covered surface, and cut into 2-inch ovals.

Preparation of topping:

Rinse and drain soaked pine nuts. Whisk together cinnamon and agave until well coated. Pour over pine nuts.

Assembly:

Scoop 1 Tbsp. of topping mixture onto each cookie and lightly press in. Dehydrate at 110° for 8 hours.

Makes 16 cookies.

Chocolate Truffles

For chocolate lovers around the world, raw cacao offers high-energy health benefits that are guilt free and a great alternative to milk chocolates and other highly processed and chemical-laden varieties. Raw cacao is rich in magnesium, calcium, and mood-enhancing agents that set off the "love reactors" in the brain.

These truffles are all easy to prepare and can be saved for up to 21 days in the refrigerator. One way to enhance the healing benefit of these high-energy treats is to add superfoods to balance the chocolate and add additional nutritional value to each bite. For example, add 2 Tbsp. SuperGreens, spirulina, or maca-root powder.

— BLOOD-ORANGE TRUFFLES —

2 cups room-temperature Chocolate Base (page 137)   1 tsp. cinnamon
½ cup blood-orange juice or tea   1 tsp. Himalayan salt
½ cup agave nectar

Blend juice, nectar, cinnamon, and salt into a thick syrup. Pour Chocolate Base into small cups ⅓ full. Fill in another ⅓ with orange mixture. Refrigerate 1 hour. Enjoy! Makes 16 truffles.

— MINT-CACAO TRUFFLES —

2 cups chilled Chocolate Base (page 137)   ½ cup agave nectar
2 cups fresh mint   ½ cup young Thai coconut water
1 cup pine nuts   1 cup young Thai coconut flesh
1 Tbsp. vanilla extract or 4 vanilla beans

Blend all ingredients (except chocolate) until rich and creamy. Place in a squeeze bottle. Take chilled Chocolate Base and scoop out 2-inch balls; then press flat into squares. Pull up corners into peaks and fill with mixture. Refrigerate 1 hour. Makes 16 truffles.

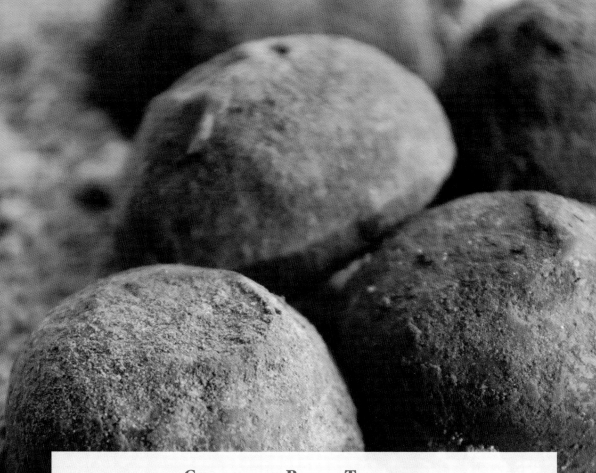

— CHOCOLATE PECAN TRUFFLES —

2 cups chilled Chocolate Base (page 137)
2½ cups coarsely ground pecan pieces
2 Tbsp. cinnamon
1 tsp. Himalayan salt

Combine pecans, cinnamon, and salt in a food processor and pulse into a fine topping. Using an ice-cream scoop or spoon, scoop out 2-Tbsp. pieces of base and form into 2-inch balls with your hands by rolling in a circular pattern, and then roll in the pecan mixture. Refrigerate 1 hour and enjoy!

Makes 16 truffles.

Luscious Cakes

When cakes are made with healthful, raw living ingredients, they can be enjoyed as a guilt-free delicious meal any time of day or night! You'll love their flavor and texture—as well as the knowledge that they're high in protein, vitamins, minerals, and superfoods.

— BACIO CRÈME CAKE —

FILLING:

4 cups macadamia nuts (soaked 8 hours)
2 cups agave nectar
3 Tbsp. raw cacao

1 tsp. Himalayan salt
5 cups young Thai coconut water
2 Tbsp. vanilla extract or 4 vanilla beans

CRUST:

2 cups hazelnuts
1 pinch Himalayan salt
½ tsp. nutmeg

1 tsp. cinnamon
½ cup agave nectar

Crust preparation:

Begin by placing hazelnuts in a food processor and pulse to a fine powder. Add remaining ingredients until a crust-like ball forms. Remove, and spread about ½-inch thick into a 10-inch springform pan.

Assembly:

Rinse and drain soaked macadamia nuts. In a high-power blender, combine all filling ingredients, except for cacao. Blend well. Pour half of the mixture on top of the crust. Add cacao to remaining mixture and blend well. Pour over non-cacao mixture. Freeze at least 6 hours. Cut into pie pieces and serve.

Makes 10 slices.

— CHOCOLATE CAKE —

4 cups Nut-Flour Base (use almonds—see page 137)
1 tsp. cinnamon
2 cups Chocolate Sauce (page 134)
1 Tbsp. vanilla extract or 5 vanilla beans
4 Tbsp. cold-pressed extra-virgin olive oil

Process all ingredients in a food processor until dough ball forms. Press into a 10-inch springform cake mold. Place in dehydrator at 115° for 4 hours, or freeze 1 hour. Decorate, and serve chilled.

Makes 10 slices.

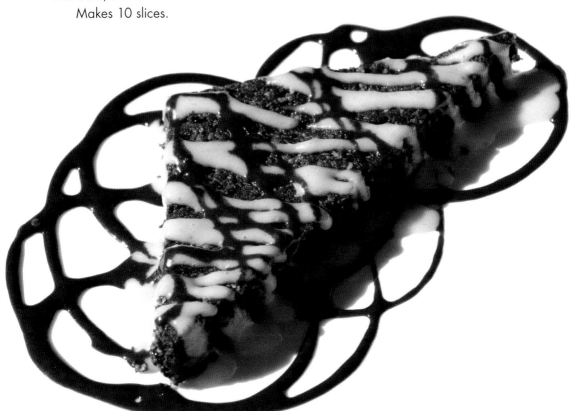

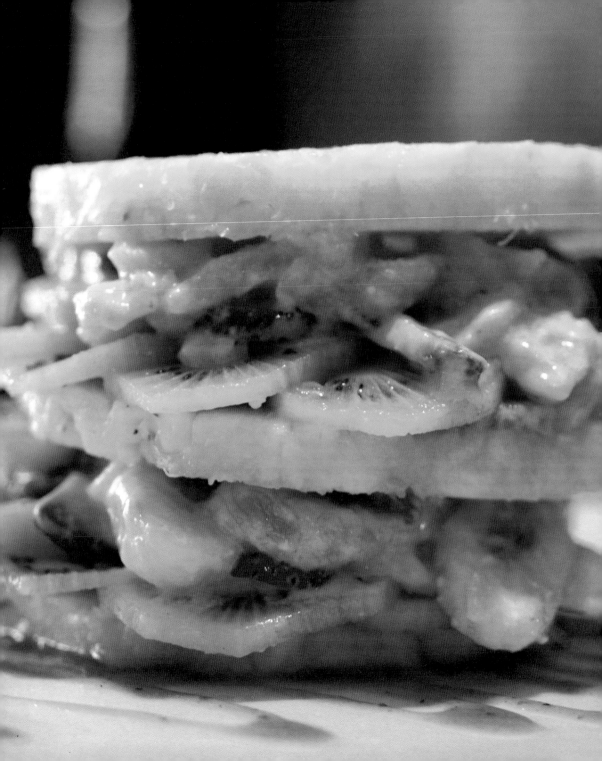

— Pineapple Sandwich —

1 small to midsize pineapple
1 cup Vanilla Sauce (page 135)
8 large strawberries

1 large Hass avocado
1 banana
2 kiwis

Begin by cutting pineapple into ½-inch-thick rounds. Skin kiwi and cut into ¼-inch-thick rounds. Set pineapple and kiwi aside. Cut strawberries into ¼-inch rounds. Chop banana and avocado into ½-inch-thick pieces. In a medium-sized mixing bowl, combine Vanilla Sauce, strawberries, avocado, and banana, and toss well. Then begin by layering pineapple, kiwi, and ¼ cup fruit mixture. Repeat, and top with one final layer of pineapple.

Pies

Pies are one of the easiest ways to introduce someone to living cuisine. Make one to last all week (although it may be irresistible and vanish sooner!). I (Jenny) eat mine for snacks and breakfast because they're high in protein. You will need to prepare a Pecan Pie Crust (see below) for all the recipes in this section except the Banana-Butter Pie and Apple Pie.

— Pecan Pie Crust —

2 cups soaked pecan pieces
1 cup agave nectar
½ tsp. cinnamon

½ tsp. sea salt
½ tsp. vanilla extract or 1 vanilla bean

Combine all ingredients in a food processor. Process until a dough ball forms. Dough may be frozen for later use or dehydrated in an 8-inch pie mold and saved. Dehydrate 12 hours at 115° for optimal results, or freeze crust for one hour before filling. Makes 1 pie crust.

— PEAR PIE —

The delicious golden hues of a perfectly ripe pear were inspiration enough for this delightful recipe. A flavorful blend of fresh fruit, cinnamon, vanilla, and of course, love, this pie makes a great dessert for any time of the day! Be sure to share with family and friends, as it's entirely too good to keep to yourself! Place entire pie into refrigerator for 1 hour or into dehydrator for 2 hours at 110° to set.

4 fresh pears, diced
1 Tbsp. vanilla extract or 2 vanilla beans
4 Tbsp. Vanilla Sauce (page 135)

1 tsp. nutmeg
1 tsp. cinnamon

Combine all ingredients (except Vanilla Sauce) in a food processor and pulse until thick and chunky. In a large bowl, add mixture to Vanilla Sauce and fold together. Fill into pie crust. Makes one 8-inch pie.

— MIXED-BERRY PIE —

Berries are packed with antioxidants and abounding with flavor. Strawberries and blackberries work best with this recipe, although your local farmer may surprise you with a fresh pick of several other varieties. Berries are good for your heart and your overall well-being, so dig in to this recipe without reservation . . . and enjoy!

4 cups fresh mixed berries
1 cup raspberries
1 cup agave nectar

1 tsp. psyllium husk
1 tsp. sea salt

Blend raspberries in a blender. Add agave, sea salt, and psyllium. Blend until thick. Chop mixed berries, and combine with raspberry mixture in a bowl. Add to pie crust and chill 1 hour. Remove from freezer and slice into pieces to enjoy. Garnish with Vanilla Sauce (page 135) and Chocolate Sauce (page 134) for plating and additional flavor. Leftovers may be refrigerated for up to 3 days. Makes one 8-inch pie.

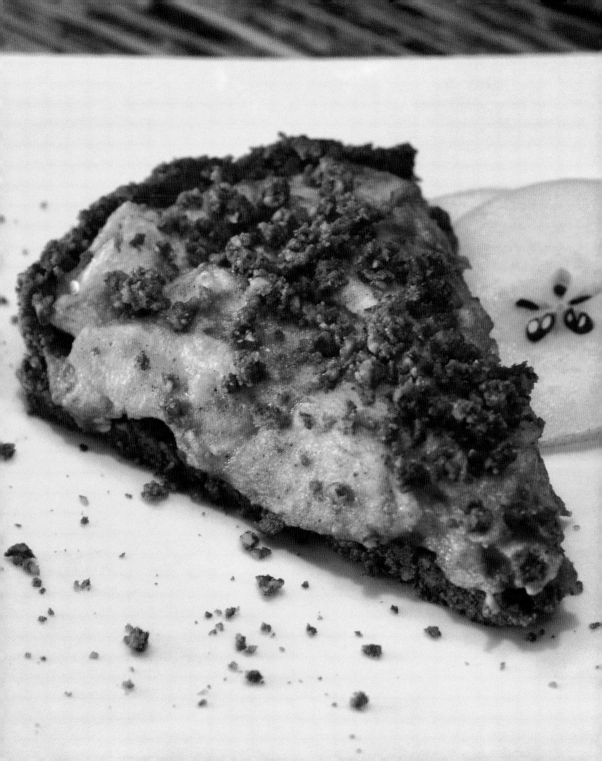

— APPLE PIE —

Apple pie is a classic American dessert, and many 118 customers have raved that this recipe rivals the best of the best. It makes an excellent breakfast pie that's delicious and healthful. For best results, enjoy warm, fresh out of the dehydrator and drizzled with caramel. This treat goes quickly, so make sure you have plenty on hand to serve your hungry friends!

PIE CRUST:
> 2 cups walnuts (soaked 4 hours)
> 1 cup agave nectar
> ½ Tbsp. cinnamon
> ½ tsp. sea salt

PIE FILLING:
> 4 apples, cored and sliced thin
> 1 cup agave nectar
> 1 Tbsp. cinnamon

Preparation of crust:

Rinse and drain soaked walnuts. Combine all ingredients in a food processor and process until dough mixture forms. Press out flat about ½-inch thick over nonstick drying sheet or into 8-inch pie mold, and dehydrate at 110° for 2 hours.

Preparation of filling:

In a large mixing bowl, combine all ingredients and mix well using a large spatula. Place in dehydrator, and dehydrate at 110° for 2 hours.

Assembly:

Remove crust and filling from dehydrator. Fill crust with apple mixture using a wooden spoon; or spread about 1-inch thick over flat crust, and garnish with your choice of 3 Tbsp. Caramel Sauce or Vanilla Sauce (page 135).

Makes one 8-inch pie.

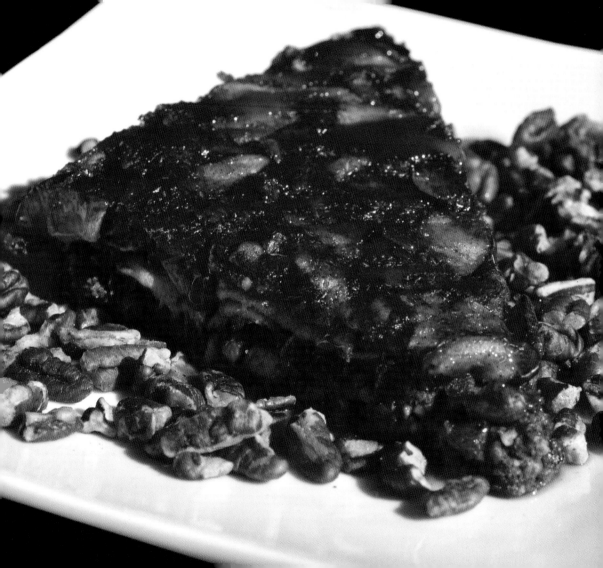

— PUMPKIN PIE —

This is a holiday classic that won't add to your waistline! Enjoy this recipe all winter long, and make sure to take it with you when joining friends at potlucks and parties. They are sure to remark that it's the freshest-tasting pumpkin pie they've ever enjoyed!

4 cups chopped pumpkin	3 Tbsp. psyllium husk	1 tsp. sea salt
1 Tbsp. pumpkin-pie spice	1 Tbsp. vanilla extract or 4 vanilla beans	
1 tsp. cinnamon	4 Tbsp. cold-pressed extra-virgin olive oil	

Blend all ingredients (except psyllium) until creamy. Add psyllium husk. Blend until thick. Add filling to crust and leave 4 hours to set in the freezer. Remove, and slice into pieces. Garnish with Caramel Sauce and Vanilla Sauce (page 135) for a decadent dessert. Leftovers may be refrigerated for up to 3 days. Makes one 8-inch pie.

— BANANA-BUTTER PIE —

This rich and creamy frozen pie can be enjoyed any time of the day and is a great use for overripe bananas. The recipe is quick and easy to prepare and lasts up to 10 days in the freezer.

2 cups banana (about 4 midsize bananas)	1 tsp. pumpkin-pie spice
16 oz. almond butter	1 tsp. vanilla extract
1 cup agave nectar	1 tsp. Himalayan salt
1 Tbsp. cinnamon	½ cup crushed almonds, for garnish (optional)

In a high-powered blender, combine all ingredients (except almonds) and blend well. Pour into a 10-inch springform pan. Sprinkle with crushed almonds for garnish, and let set in freezer 4 hours. Makes 10 slices.

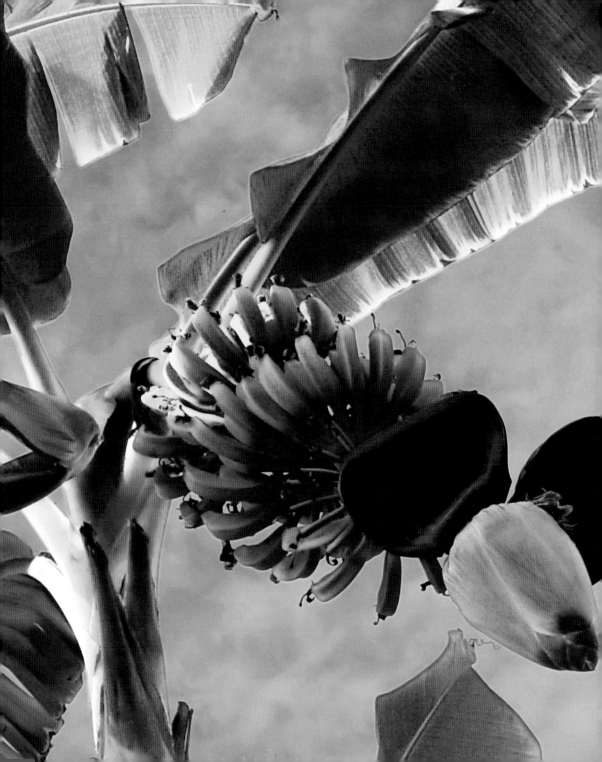

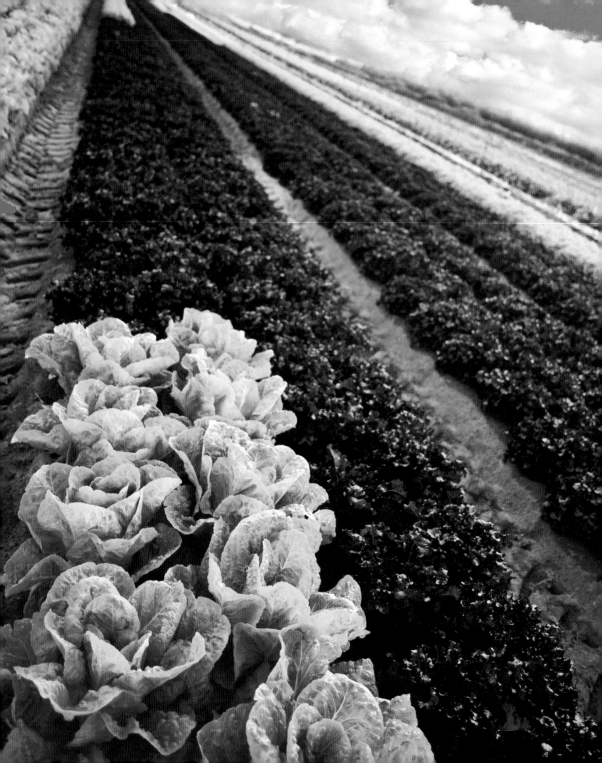

Afterword

Whether you incorporate some raw living food into your daily meals or decide to embrace a living-foods diet 100 percent, you'll experience great benefits from this healthful way of eating. Raw vegetables, fruits, nuts, and grains offer you increased energy, vitality, health, beauty, and intuition; as well as other positive experiences.

You may feel inspired to grow your own herb, fruit, or vegetable garden. With a garden, you'll eat the freshest of produce and have intimate dealings with Mother Nature. We find that our food cravings are reduced when we're handling fruits and vegetables during the preparation of raw living cuisine.

We hope that you'll view the recipes in this book as a wonderful springboard for you to develop your own unique creations, whether in food or in other areas of life. Explore and experiment with the entire palette of rainbow colors in the fresh-food world, as well as with every dream and desire you have!

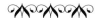

References

Agren, J. J.; Törmälä, M. L.; Nenonen, M. T.; Hänninen, O. O. "Fatty acid composition of erythrocyte, platelet, and serum lipids in strict vegans." *Lipids*, April 1995; vol. 30, pp. 365–369.

Agren, J. J.; Tvrzicka, E.; Nenonen, M. T.; Helve, T., Hänninen, O. "Divergent changes in serum sterols during a strict uncooked vegan diet in patients with rheumatoid arthritis." *British Journal of Nutrition*, February 2001; vol. 85, pp. 137–139.

Boutenko, V., *Green for Life*. Ashland, OR: Raw Family Publishing, 2005.

Campbell, T. C., and Campbell, T. M. *The China Study: The Most Comprehensive Study of Nutrition Ever Conducted and the Startling Implications for Diet, Weight Loss and Long-Term Health*. Dallas, TX: BenBella Books, Inc., 2006.

Cousens, G. *Rainbow Green Live-Food Cuisine*. Berkeley, CA: North Atlantic Books, 2003.

Donaldson, M. S. "Metabolic vitamin B12 status on a mostly raw vegan diet with follow-up using tablets, nutritional yeast, or probiotic supplements." *Annals of Nutrition and Metabolism*, 2000; vol. 44, pp. 229–234.

Donaldson, M. S.; Speight, N.; Loomis, S. "Fibromyalgia syndrome improved using a mostly raw vegetarian diet: an observational study." *BMC Complementary and Alternative Medicine*, 2001; vol. 1, p. 7.

Douglass, J. M.; Rasgon, I. M.; Fleiss, P. M.; Schmidt, R. D.; Peters, S. N.; Abelmann, E. A. "Effects of a raw food diet on hypertension and obesity." *Southern Medical Journal*, July 1985; vol. 78, pp. 841–844.

Ganss, C.; Schlechtriemen, M.; Klimek, J. "Dental erosions in subjects living on a raw food diet." *Caries Research*, 1999; vol. 33, pp. 74–80.

Hänninen, O.; Kaartinen, K.; Rauma, A.; Nenonen, M.; Törrönen, R.; Häkkinen, S.; Adlercreutz, H.; Laakso , J. "Antioxidants in vegan diet and rheumatic disorders." *Toxicology*, November 30, 2000; vol. 155, pp. 45–53.

Hänninen, O.; Nenonen, M.; Ling, W. H.; Li, D. S.; Sihvonen, L. "Effects of eating an uncooked vegetable diet for 1 week." *Appetite*, December 1992; vol. 19, pp. 243–254.

Hänninen, O.; Rauma, A. L.; Kaartinen, K.; Nenonen, M. "Vegan diet in physiological health promotion." *Acta Physiologica Hungarica*, 1999; vol. 86, pp.171–180.

Kaartinen, K.; Lammi, K.; Hypen, M.; Nenonen, M.; Hänninen, O.; Rauma, A. L. "Vegan diet alleviates fibromyalgia symptoms." *Scandinavian Journal of Rheumatology*, 2000; vol. 29, pp. 308–313.

Koebnick, C.; Strassner, C.; Hoffmann, I.; Leitzmann, C. "Consequences of a long-term raw food diet on body weight and menstruation: results of a questionnaire survey." *Annals of Nutrition and Metabolism*, 1999; vol. 43, pp. 69–79.

Nenonen, M. T.; Helve, T. A.; Rauma, A. L.; Hänninen, O. O. "Uncooked, lactobacilli-rich, vegan food and rheumatoid arthritis." *British Journal of Rheumatology*, March 1998; vol. 37, pp. 274–281.

Patenaude, F., *The Raw Secrets: The Raw Food Diet in the Real World*. Montreal: FredericPatenaude.com, 2006.

Peltonen, R.; Ling, W. H.; Hänninen, O.; Eerola, E. "An uncooked vegan diet shifts the profile of human fecal microflora: computerized analysis of direct stool sample gas-liquid chromatography profiles of bacterial cellular fatty acids." *Applied and Environmental Microbiology*, November 1992; vol. 58, pp. 3660–3666.

Peltonen, R.; Nenonen, M.; Helve, T.; Hänninen, O.; Toivanen, P.; Eerola, E. "Faecal microbial flora and disease activity in rheumatoid arthritis during a vegan diet." *British Journal of Rheumatology*, January 1997; vol. 36, pp. 64–68.

Rauma A. L.; Nenonen, M.; Helve, T.; Hänninen, O. "Effect of a strict vegan diet on energy and nutrient intakes by Finnish rheumatoid patients." *European Journal of Clinical Nutrition*, October 1993; vol. 47, pp. 747–749.

Rauma, A. L.; Törrönen, R.; Hänninen, O.; Mykkänen, H. "Vitamin B-12 status of long-term adherents of a strict uncooked vegan diet ('living food diet') is compromised." *The Journal of Nutrition*, October 1995; vol. 125, pp. 2511–2515.

Rauma, A. L.; Törrönen, R.; Hänninen, O.; Verhagen, H.; Mykkänen, H. "Antioxidant status in long-term adherents to a strict uncooked vegan diet." *American Journal of Clinical Nutrition*, December 1995; vol. 62, pp. 1221–1227.

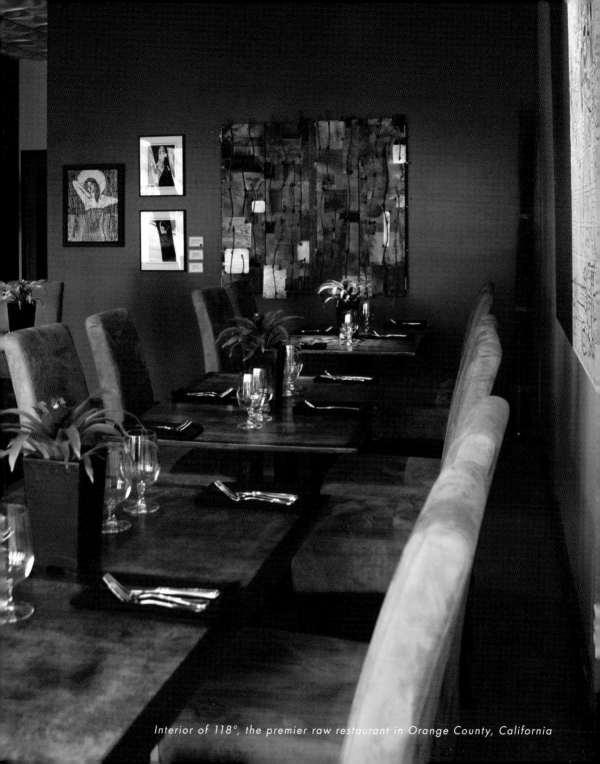

Interior of 118°, the premier raw restaurant in Orange County, California

About the Authors

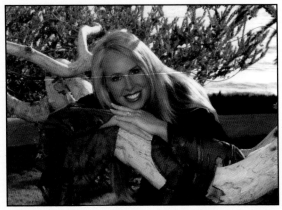

www.photographybycheryl.com

Doreen Virtue is a metaphysician and former psychotherapist who specialized in treating eating disorders. She has written four previous books about diet and eating: the best-selling *The Yo-Yo Diet Syndrome, Losing Your Pounds of Pain, Constant Craving,* and *Eating in the Light.* She has appeared on *Oprah,* CNN, *The View,* and other programs worldwide.

Doreen has been a vegan since 1996, eating 80 to 90 percent raw food. She first tried prepared raw food at Juliano's Organica café in San Francisco in 1999, right before giving a workshop. She noticed a huge increase in her energy and psychic abilities during the workshop, which she credited to the raw food. She continued to eat it at Organica during her regular visits to San Francisco, where she gave psychic readings at the Palo Alto Unity Church. Doreen went 100 percent raw for a year, from 2007 to 2008, and today continues her vegan diet with mostly raw living food.

Website: **www.AngelTherapy.com**

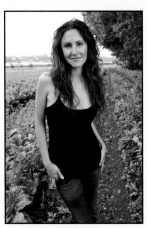

Curtis Bailey

Jenny Ross is a raw-food chef and the CEO of Creative Blend, a company that produces and distributes raw-food meals called Jenny's Raw and Organic at health-food stores. She's the owner and culinary creator of 118°, the premier Orange County raw restaurant, which is continually filled with happy customers from all walks of life. A former model, Jenny discovered raw food in 1999 in her own personal quest to enjoy vibrant health, and she learned how to prepare it by studying with raw-food chefs from around the world. Afterward, she realized her passion to share the journey of healthful eating with others and began working with living foods professionally in the year 2000.

Jenny regularly gives speeches and interviews about raw foods and teaches raw-food-preparation classes. She's appeared on *G Word* on the Discovery Channel; Travel Channel's *Taste of America* program; and Channels 5, 7, and 9 in Los Angeles. Jenny was honored as a Hot 25 influential business leader in Orange County in 2008 by *OC Metro,* and was dubbed the "Sexiest Chef" in Orange County in 2007 by *Riviera* magazine.

Website: **www.shop118degrees.com**

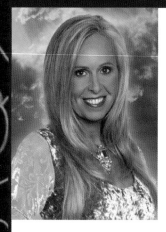

Hay House Titles of Related Interest

YOU CAN HEAL YOUR LIFE, *the movie*, starring Louise L. Hay & Friends
(available as a 1-DVD program and an expanded 2-DVD set)
Watch the trailer at: **www.LouiseHayMovie.com**

THE SHIFT, *the movie,* starring Dr. Wayne W. Dyer
(available as a 1-DVD program and an expanded 2-DVD set)
Watch the trailer at: **www.DyerMovie.com**

THE ART OF EXTREME SELF-CARE: *Transform Your Life One Month at a Time,*
by Cheryl Richardson

THE CORE BALANCE DIET: *4 Weeks to Boost Your Metabolism and Lose Weight for Good,*
by Marcelle Pick, R.N.P., with Genevieve Morgan

GREEN MADE EASY: *The Everyday Guide for Transitioning to a Green Lifestyle*,
by Chris Prelitz

RECIPES FOR HEALTH BLISS: *Using NatureFoods & Lifestyle Choices to Rejuvenate Your Body & Life,* by Susan Smith Jones, Ph.D.

TO SERVE WITH LOVE: *Simple, Scrumptious Dishes from the Skinny to the Sinful,*
by Carnie Wilson

VEGETARIAN MEALS FOR PEOPLE-ON-THE-GO: *101 Quick & Easy Recipes,*
by Vimala Rodgers

THE VITAMIN D REVOLUTION: *How the Power of This Amazing Vitamin Can Change Your Life,* by Soram Khalsa, M.D.

All of the above are available at your local bookstore,
or may be ordered by contacting Hay House (see last page).

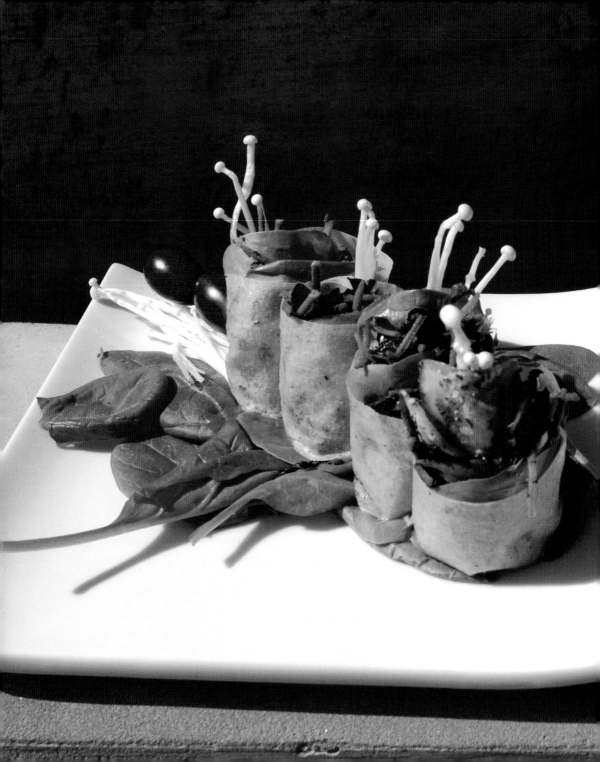

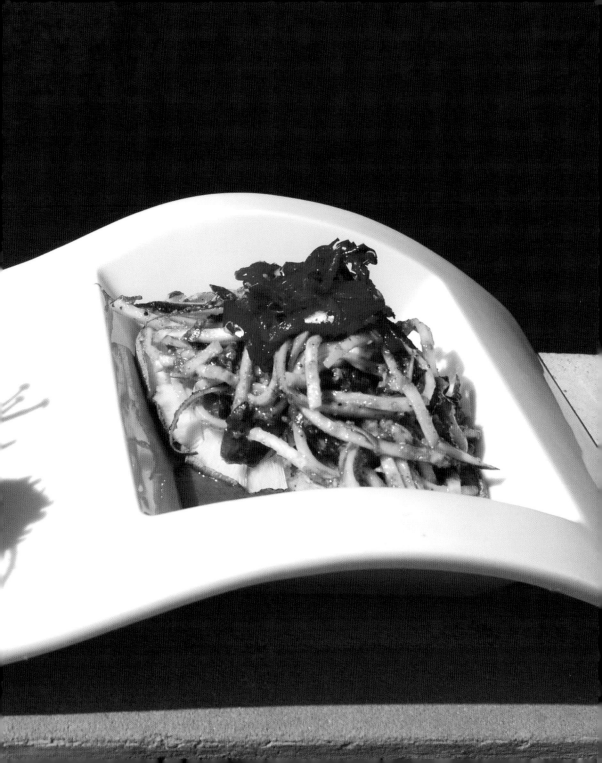

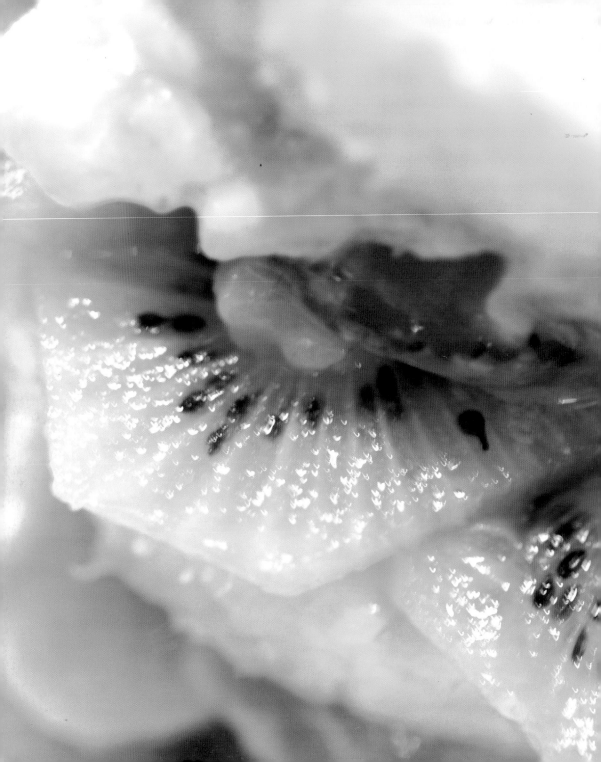